CONCISE CARDIOVASCULAR DISEASE BOARD REVIEW

KEY CONCEPTS FOR SUCCESS

Thomas J. Sawyer, MD, FACC
Clinical Assistant Professor of Medicine
University of Washington Medical Center
Staff Cardiologist, Summit Cardiology
Seattle, Washington

cardiotext.
PUBLISHING
Minneapolis, Minnesota

Cardiotext Publishing, LLC
3405 W. 44th Street
Minneapolis, Minnesota 55410
USA

www.cardiotextpublishing.com

Any updates to this book may be found at: www.cardiotextpublishing.com/assorted-cardiology/
concise-cardiovascular-disease-board-review

Comments, inquiries, and requests for bulk sales can be directed to the publisher at: info@cardiotext-
publishing.com.

Library of Congress Control Number: 2018939870

ISBN: 978-1-942909-23-1

eISBN: 978-1-942909-28-6

Printed in the United States of America

 2 3 4 5 6 7 22 21 20 19

Dedication

To my Mom and Dad.

Thank you for making everything possible.

Table of Contents

Preface

Concise Cardiovascular Disease Board Review is intended to completely summarize the key concepts necessary for success on the ABIM cardiovascular disease examination with an emphasis on ACC/AHA guideline recommendations. Several excellent board review texts are currently available which are very long and include detailed information on clinical trials, pathophysiology, and basic science. These are important details to know, but not directly relevant to the ABIM exam. The intent of this book is to strip away the background information that is not tested and focus exclusively on high yield material geared specifically for the ABIM exam, allowing users to maximize their study time.

This has particular relevance in light of the new ABIM pathway allowing a "Knowledge Check-in" recertification every two years. This will require more focused review over a shorter period of time, which is a specific intent of this text. When the open book option for the 10-year "long form" assessment begins this book will be an ideal resource for an exam of that style as well.

Content of the book is based directly upon the ABIM Cardiovascular Disease examination blueprint (https://www.abim.org/~/media/ABIM%20Public/Files/pdf/exam-blueprints/certification/cardiovascular-disease.pdf) and chapters will be ordered from the most to least emphasized topics according to the blueprint.

Though the physical examination chapter is towards the end of the text, it should be a point of emphasis in your study. The majority of board exam question stems are long and include detailed physical examination findings. Recognizing the findings and conditions they represent will be invaluable for the examination and is necessary in order to move quickly enough to complete the examination in the allotted time.

For those preparing for initial certification, the ECG portion of the exam is equally important. The gold standard for ECG board preparation remains *The Complete Guide to ECGs* by James H. O'Keefe Jr., et al., and therefore, a formal ECG section is not included in this text.

Any ECGs used in this text that are not original are sourced from *Podrid's Real-World ECGs* and have been graciously provided by Cardiotext Publishing.

Several review texts are available in question and answer format though none specifically recreate the format typically seen on the boards. The best resource for "board style" questions is the medical knowledge section of the ABIM website which offers multiple learning modules covering various topics, each with 30 board style questions and explanations of the answer. These can be found through the Physician Portal on the ABIM website (https://portal .abim.org/). Completion of these modules also earns credit necessary for Maintenance of Certification.

Preparing for boards can be a stressful and time-consuming process. However, it is also an opportunity to expand and solidify your knowledge base. My hope is this book will make your preparation a little easier. Despite the stress, boards are an exciting time and represent the culmination of years of hard work and effort. Good luck and enjoy the process!

CHAPTER 1

ACUTE CORONARY SYNDROME

ANTIPLATELET/ANTICOAGULANT STRATEGIES

All patients receive aspirin, P2Y12 inhibitor, and anticoagulant

- ASA 162–325 mg initially / 75–100 mg daily
- P2Y12 inhibitor
  - Plavix 300–600 mg load / 75 mg daily
  - Ticagrelor 180 mg load / 90 mg bid
    - ASA maintenance dose should be no greater than 81 mg daily with ticagrelor
  - Prasugrel 60 mg load / 10 mg bid
    - Only given in the cath lab after decision made for PCI
    - Contraindicated age > 75 or Hx CVA / TIA
- Anticoagulants
  - Heparin 60–80 U/kg bolus / 18 U/kg gtt goal aPTT 50–70
  - Enoxaparin 1 mg/kg
  - Bivalirudin

- 2B/3A inhibitor
  - Only used for patients not pretreated with P2Y12 inhibitor
  - Eptifibatide 180 mcg/kg IV bolus over 1–2 min / 2 mcg/kg/min gtt

UA/NSTEMI— INVASIVE VS. CONSERVATIVE APPROACH

- TIMI score
  - Age > 65
  - 3+ cardiac RFs
    - Family history of premature CAD
      - < 55-year-old male / < 65-year-old female
    - HTN
    - Hyperlipidemia
    - DM
    - Tobacco abuse
  - Known CAD (any lesion > 50%)
  - ASA use in the last 7 days
  - 2 or more anginal episodes in preceding 24 hours
  - ST segment deviation
  - Elevated troponin
  - ≥ 3 = high risk
    - Invasive strategy preferred (cath 4–24 hours after admission)
  - 0–2 = low risk
    - Consider conservative management

- UA/NSTEMI – Invasive strategy
  - Coronary angiography should be 4–24 hours after admission → no difference in outcomes first 24 hours

- UA/NSTEMI – Conservative strategy
  - **NOTE**: Only difference in anticoagulation / antiplatelet strategy between invasive and conservative strategy is that prasugrel and bivalirudin are not indicated for a conservative approach
  - Fondaparinux can be used as an anticoagulant (contraindicated for invasive strategy due to increased risk of catheter thrombosis)
  - Duration of therapy in conservative strategy
    - Heparin × 48 hours
    - 2B/3A inhibitor × 48 hours
    - Enoxaparin / fondaparinux used duration of hospitalization (up to 8 days)
    - For NSTEMI, P2Y12 inhibitor indicated for **12 months** even if BMS or no PCI
- **No indication for PCI in spontaneous dissection →** typically treated medically

STEMI

- Presentation < 12 hours after symptom onset → always reperfuse
- 12–24 hours → reperfuse if CHF, VT, persistent symptoms
- Presentation > 24 hours after symptom onset, no clear indication for reperfusion unless presenting with cardiogenic shock and can be reperfused within 18 hours of the onset of shock symptoms

- PCI vs. lytics
  - In general, PCI preferred if available within the time goals below:
    - PCI within 90 minutes of **first medical contact** (not symptoms) or 120 minutes if being transferred to a PCI-capable facility
    - If primary PCI unavailable, goal for lytic administration is 30 minutes from **first medical contact**
  - Antiplatelet / anticoagulant strategy for PCI identical to UA/NSTEMI invasive approach

- Fibrinolytics (streptokinase, alteplase, reteplase, tenecteplase)
  - Coadminister
    - ASA 325 mg
    - Plavix **300 mg** (75 mg if > 75 years old)
    - UFH or enoxaparin
    - **No** 2B/3A with thrombolytics
  - Absolute contraindications
    - Hx intracranial hemorrhage
    - Ischemic CVA within last 3 months
    - Closed head or facial trauma within last 3 months
    - Active bleeding
    - Aortic dissection
    - Intracranial lesion / malignancy
  - Transfer to PCI-capable facility after administering fibrinolytics
    - Successful reperfusion and EF > 40% → continue standard medical Rx
    - EF < 40% → cath
    - Rescue PCI for < 50% ST resolution at 90 minutes, ventricular arrhythmia, persistent ischemic symptoms

POST-INFARCT COMPLICATIONS

○ Ventricular septal defect
   ● Exam is usually diagnostic
      • Shock with signs of biventricular failure
      • Loud, holosystolic murmur that radiates widely +/– precordial thrill
   ● Surgical emergency
   ● Short-acting vasodilator (nitroprusside) reduces afterload and L → R shunt preoperatively

○ LV aneurysm
   ● Involves all layers of the myocardium (wide neck on echo)

○ Pseudoaneurysm
   ● LV rupture contained by pericardium (narrow neck on echo)
   ● Surgical emergency

○ Papillary muscle rupture
   ● Posteromedial most common – blood supply from RCA only
   ● Anterior with blood supply from LAD / Cx
   ● Surgical emergency
   ● IABP, vasodilator, diuretics for stabilization preoperatively

○ VT / VF **> 48 hours post-MI**
   ● Indication for ICD
   ● < 48 hours → treat symptomatically

○ Post-MI pericarditis
   ● High-dose ASA (600 mg q6h)
   ● Colchicine 0.6 mg bid
   ● All NSAIDs except ASA contraindicated post-MI

- Dressler's syndrome
  - Acute pericarditis 1–8 weeks post-MI associated with fever, malaise, leukocytosis, elevated inflammatory markers
- Advise women to stop HRT post-MI

REFERENCES

1. Dash D. Current status of antiplatelet therapy in acute coronary syndrome. *Cardiovasc Hematol Agents Med Chem.* 2015;13(1):40–49.

2. Amsterdam EA, Wenger NK, Brindis RG, et al. 2014 AHA/ACC guideline for the management of patients with non ST elevation acute coronary syndromes: A report of the American College of Cardiology/American Heart Association Task Force on Practice Guidelines. *Circulation.* 2014;130:2354–2394.

3. O'Gara PT, Kushner FG, Ascheim DD, et al. 2013 ACCF/AHA guideline for the management of ST elevation myocardial infarction: A report of the American College of Cardiology Foundation/American Heart Association Task Force on Practice Guidelines. *Circulation.* 2013;127(4):e362–e425.

4. Aksoy O, Tuzcu EM. Chapter 42: Complications of myocardial infarction. In: Griffin BP, Kapadia SR, Rimmerman CM. *The Cleveland clinic cardiology board review.* 2nd ed. Philadelphia: Lippincott Williams & Wilkins; 2013:607–626.

5. Ibanez B, James S, Agewall S, et al. 2017 ESC Guidelines for the management of acute myocardial infarction in patients presenting with ST-segment elevation: The Task Force for the management of acute myocardial infarction in patients presenting with ST-segment elevation of the European Society of Cardiology. *Eur Heart J.* 2018;39(2):119–177. https://doi.org/10.1093/eurheartj/ehx393

CHAPTER 2

CHRONIC CAD

ANGINA DEFINITION

1. Discomfort in chest, jaw, shoulder, back, arm, epigastrium
2. Aggravated by exertion and / or emotional stress
3. Relieved by rest and / or nitroglycerin

○ 3/3 features = typical angina

○ 2/3 features = atypical angina

○ 0 or 1 feature = noncardiac

CCS ANGINA CLASSIFICATION

I: No angina with ordinary activity. Angina only with strenuous, rapid, or prolonged exertion

II: Slight limitation of ordinary activity

○ Angina after > 2 blocks / > 1 flight of stairs

III: Marked limitation of ordinary activity

○ Angina after 1–2 blocks / < 1 flight of stairs

IV: Inability to carry out any physical activity without angina or angina occurring at rest

PRETEST PROBABILITY OF CAD

> 90% = High pretest probability of CAD
10%–90% = Intermediate
< 10% = Low

- All patients at intermediate pretest probability are candidates for stress testing

- High pretest probability patients with classic symptoms are appropriate to go directly to coronary angiography, though noninvasive imaging is appropriate depending on the clinical scenario

General rules for determining pretest probability:

- MEN
  - 40 years old with non-cardiac or atypical angina = intermediate pretest probability
  - 40 years old with typical angina = high probability

- WOMEN
  - 50 years old with atypical angina = intermediate pretest probability
  - 50 years old with typical angina = high pretest probability
  - < 50 years old with typical angina = intermediate probablity

STRESS TESTING

- Exercise is always the modality of choice unless patient unable to exercise, LBBB, or paced rhythm
  - LBBB / paced rhythm → increased likelihood of artifactual septal defects / WMA → these patients should undergo pharmacologic study even if able to exercise

- All other patients capable of exercise should undergo exercise stress even if ECG uninterpretable
  - Dig effect, LVH with strain, WPW pattern
    - Must be combined with an imaging modality due to uninterpretable ECG

- Submax ETT OK 4–6 days post-MI for prognosis, activity prescription, evaluation of medical therapy

- Symptom limited ETT OK 14–21 days post-MI

- Exercise treadmill test
  - Test of choice for anyone with an interpretable ECG capable of exercise
  - Exception is patients with hx of CABG → always include imaging
  - Indications to terminate exercise
    - ST elevation / SBP drop > 10 mmHg / intolerable angina / VT / BP > 250/115

- Duke Treadmill Score (DTS)
  - Exercise time (min) – 5 × ST deviation (mm) – 4 × angina index (0 = none, 1 = non-limiting, 2 = reason for terminating test)
  - ≥ +5 = low-risk DTS
  - +4 to –10 = intermediate-risk DTS
  - –11 = high-risk DTS

- Stress echocardiogram
  - Dobutamine can be used as a stress agent if unable to exercise

- Myocardial perfusion imaging
  - Exercise stress, dobutamine or vasodilators
    - Adenosine → nonselective A2A inhibitor
      - 140 mcg/kg/min × 5–6 minutes / radiotracer at 2–3 minutes
    - Regadenoson → selective A2A inhibitor
      - 0.4 mg injection over 10 seconds / radiotracer at 1 minute
    - Dipyridamole → inhibits adenosine reuptake
      - 0.56 mg/kg/min × 4 minutes / radiotracer at 7–9 minutes
  - Radiotracers
    - SPECT
      - Technetium–99m, 140 KeV photopeak
      - Thallium–201-80 KeV photopeak
    - PET
      - Rubidium-82, oxygen-15, nitrogen-13, carbon-11, fluorine-18
      - All have 511 KeV photopeak → greater spatial and temporal resolution than SPECT
  - Radiation dose limits
    - Nonoccupational 5 mSv/year
    - Occupational 50 mSv/year

NONINVASIVE RISK STRATIFICATION

- High risk (> 3% annual mortality rate)
  - EF < 35%
  - DTS ≤ –11
  - Angina / ECG changes at low treadmill workload
  - Fall in BP or failure to increase BP > 20/10 with exercise
  - Large or multiple perfusion defects / WMA
  - High-risk patients appropriate to go directly to coronary angiography
    - PCI considered appropriate for single vessel CAD with high-risk findings on noninvasive imaging regardless of concomitant medical therapy

- Intermediate risk (1%–3% annual mortality risk)
  - EF 35%–49%
  - DTS –11 to +4 → **Class I indication for SPECT imaging**
  - Moderate size defect on perfusion imaging

- Low risk (< 1% annual mortality risk)
  - EF ≥ 50%
  - DTS ≥ +5
  - Small perfusion defect / WMA

- Low-risk patients typically managed medically

TREATMENT OF CHRONIC ISCHEMIC HEART DISEASE

- ASA 81 mg daily in all
- Clopidogrel if ASA intolerant
  - No role for combination ASA/clopidogrel in stable CAD / stable angina alone
  - Prasugrel / ticagrelor have no indication in chronic stable CAD or stable angina alone

- Statin in all
  - Age > 75 → moderate-intensity statin
  - Age ≤ 75 → high-intensity statin
- Patients with stable angina should be treated with a **minimum** of two classes of antianginals
  - A third antianginal is appropriate with recurrent symptoms
  - Beta-blockers, nitrates first-line for stable angina
  - Calcium-channel blockers, ranolazine appropriate second-line agents
    - Neither has mortality benefit in stable CAD
- ACE/ARB has no indication in chronic stable CAD if NL LV function / NL BP / No DM

REVASCULARIZATION OF CHRONIC ISCHEMIC CAD

- Only two Class I indications for coronary angiography in stable CAD
  - Refractory angina (Class III–IV) despite optimal medical therapy
  - High-risk findings on noninvasive study
    - DTS ≤ –11 / angina / ventricular arrhythmias at low workload / BP drop with exercise
    - Reduced EF < 35%
    - Large ischemic territory (> 10%)
    - Evidence of multivessel ischemia
- Indications for CABG
  - Left main > 50%
  - 3-vessel disease (greatest benefit with EF < 50% or DM)
  - 2-vessel disease with proximal LAD and EF < 50% or ischemia on noninvasive imaging
- Preoperative management of antiplatelet agents prior to CABG

Table 2.1 Preoperative Management of Antiplatelet Agents

Agent	D/C Prior to Surgery
Clopidogrel	5 days
Prasugrel	7 days
Ticagrelor	5 days
2B/3A	4 hours
Enoxaparin	12–24 hours
Fondaparinux	24 hours
Bivalirudin	3 hours

REFERENCES

1. Campeau L. Letter: Grading of angina pectoris. *Circulation.* 1976;54:522–523.

2. Gibbons RJ, Abrams J, Chatterjee K, et al. ACC/AHA 2002 guideline update for the management of patients with chronic stable angina—summary article: A report of the American College of Cardiology/American Heart Association Task Force on Practice Guidelines (Committee on the Management of Patients With Chronic Stable Angina). *Circulation.* 2003;107:149–158.

3. Fihn SD, Gardin JM, Abrams J, et al. 2012 ACCF/AHA/ACP/AATS/PCNA/SCAI/STS guideline for the diagnosis and management of patients with stable ischemic heart disease: A report of the American College of Cardiology Foundation/American Heart Association Task Force on Practice Guidelines, and the American College of Physicians, American Association for Thoracic Surgery, Preventive Cardiovascular Nurses Association, Society for Cardiovascular Angiography and Interventions, and Society of Thoracic Surgeons. *J Am Coll Cardiol.* 2012;60:2564–2603.

4. Patel MR, Dehmer GJ, Hirshfeld JW, et al. ACCF/SCAI/STS/AATS/AHA/ASNC 2009 appropriateness criteria for coronary revascularization: A report of the American College of Cardiology Foundation Appropriateness Criteria Task Force, Society for Cardiovascular Angiography and Interventions, Society of Thoracic Surgeons, American Association for Thoracic Surgery, American Heart Association, and the American Society of Nuclear Cardiology. *Circulation.* 2009;119:1330–1352.

5. Wolk MJ, Bailey SR, Doherty JU, et al. ACCF/AHA/ASE/ASNC/ HFSA/HRS/SCAI/SCCT/SCMR/STS 2013 multimodality appropriate use criteria for the detection and risk assessment of stable ischemic heart disease: A report of the American College of Cardiology Foundation Appropriate Use Criteria Task Force, American Heart Association, American Society of Echocardiography, American Society of Nuclear Cardiology, Heart Failure Society of America, Heart Rhythm Society, Society for Cardiovascular Angiography and Interventions, Society of Cardiovascular Computed Tomography, Society for Cardiovascular Magnetic Resonance, and Society of Thoracic Surgeons. *J Am Coll Cardiol.* 2014;63(4):380–406.

6. Hillis LD, Smith PK, Anderson JL, et al. 2011 ACCF/AHA guideline for coronary artery bypass graft surgery: A report of the American College of Cardiology Foundation/American Heart Association Task Force on Practice Guidelines. *Circulation.* 2011;124:e652–e735.

7. Henzlova MJ, Duvall WL, Einstein AJ, et al. ASNC imaging guidelines for SPECT nuclear cardiology procedures: Stress, protocols, and tracers. *J Nucl Cardiol.* 2016;23:606–639.

8. Brown C, Joshi B, Faraday N, et al. Emergency cardiac surgery in patients with acute coronary syndromes: A review of the evidence and perioperative implications of medical and mechanical therapeutics. *Anesth Analg.* 2011;112(4):777–799.

CHAPTER 3

ACUTE CHF

HEART FAILURE HEMODYNAMIC PROFILES

- ○ Well-compensated (warm and dry)
  - Normal PCWP / normal cardiac index
- ○ Volume overloaded (warm and wet)
  - Elevated PCWP / normal cardiac index
  - SOB / PND / orthopnea / elevated JVP / edema / rales
  - Treatment goal: decongest / afterload reduction
- ○ Volume depleted (cold and dry)
  - Normal PCWP / low cardiac index
    - Low BP / cool extremities
    - Volume resuscitate
- ○ Cardiogenic shock (cold and wet)
  - Elevated PCWP / low cardiac index
  - SOB / PND / orthopnea / elevated JVP / edema / rales
  - Low BP / cool extremities / fatigue / confusion / end organ dysfunction
  - Treatment

- Inotropes / mechanical circulatory support to improve perfusion
- Decongest

FACTORS COMMONLY PRECIPITATING HEART FAILURE

○ Acute coronary syndrome

○ Medication noncompliance

○ Drugs
  - Negative inotropes (beta-blockers, calcium-channel blockers)
  - Salt retention (NSAIDs, steroids)

○ Arrhythmias (especially atrial fibrillation)

○ Alcohol / drug abuse

○ Pulmonary embolism

○ Hyperthyroidism / hypothyroidism

○ Infection (via cytokine release)

MEDICAL THERAPY

- ○ Diuretics are first-line therapy in treating congestion
  - ◉ Typically start with 2–2.5 times the total daily PO dose as an IV bolus
    - • Give as soon as possible → early diuretic administration associated with improved outcomes
  - ◉ Titrate diuretics as necessary to relieve congestion
    - • Diuretic effect can be enhanced either by increasing diuretic dose or adding a second agent (typically a thiazide, i.e., metolazone / chlorothiazide)
  - ◉ IV drip or multiple boluses throughout the day will improve effectiveness as sodium reabsorption will rebound once diuretic effect wears off and loop diuretics have relatively short half-life
    - • No clear advantage to bolus dosing vs. continuous infusion
- ○ Vasodilators
  - ◉ Nitroglycerin → venodilation → reduced preload
  - ◉ Nitroprusside → arterial and venodilation → reduced preload, markedly reduced afterload
    - • Indicated for HTN emergency, severe acute AI, severe MR, acute VSD

- ○ Inotropes
  - ◉ Indicated in patients unresponsive to or intolerant of vasodilators / diuretics
  - ◉ Milrinone → vasodilating inotrope
    - Phosphodiesterase inhibitor → increased cAMP → vasodilation
    - Pulmonary vasodilation / OK to use with beta-blockers
    - 0.375–0.75 mcg/kg/min
  - ◉ Dobutamine → vasodilating inotrope
    - Beta-agonist → decreased afterload (via beta-2 mediated vasodilation of vascular smooth muscle)
    - 2–5 mcg/kg/min
  - ◉ Dopamine
    - 2–5 mcg/kg/min → beta-1 → increased chronotropy
    - 5–15 mcg/kg/min → alpha-1 → vasoconstriction
  - ◉ Norepinephrine
    - Primarily alpha-1 → vasoconstriction
    - 0.01–3.0 mcg/kg/min
  - ◉ Epinephrine
    - Beta-1 / beta-2 / alpha → increased contractility and afterload
    - 0.01-0.1 mcg/kg/min
- ○ Ultrafiltration may be considered in patients with refractory volume overload (IIb indication)

REFERENCES

1. Nohria A, Lewis E, Stevenson LW. Medical management of acute heart failure. *JAMA.* 2002;287(5):628–640. (doi:10.1001/jama.287.5.628)

2. Yancy CW, Jessup M, Bozkurt B, et al. 2013 ACCF/AHA guideline for the management of heart failure: A report of the American College of Cardiology Foundation/American Heart Association Task Force on Practice Guidelines. *J Am Coll Cardiol.* 2013;62:e147–e239. (doi: 10.1016/j.jacc.2013.05.019)

3. Yancy CW, Jessup M, Bozkurt B, et al. 2017 ACC/AHA/HFSA focused update of the 2013 ACCF/AHA guideline for the management of heart failure: A report of the American College of Cardiology/American Heart Association Task Force on Clinical Practice Guidelines and the Heart Failure Society of America. *J Am Coll Cardiol.* 2017;70:776–803. (doi: 10.1016/j.jacc.2017.04.025)

4. Ponikowski P, Voors A, Anker S, et al. 2016 ESC Guidelines for the diagnosis and treatment of acute and chronic heart failure: The Task Force for the diagnosis and treatment of acute and chronic heart failure of the European Society of Cardiology (ESC). Developed with the special contribution of the Heart Failure Association (HFA) of the ESC. *Eur Heart J.* 2016;37(27):2129–2200. (doi: 10.1093/eurheartj/ehw128)

5. Lindenfeld J, Albert NM, Boehmer JP, et al. Executive Summary: HFSA 2010 comprehensive heart failure practice guideline. *J Card Fail.* 2010;16:475–539. (doi: 10.1016/j.cardfail.2010.04.004)

6. Parks KA, Januzzi JL. Chapter 14: Diagnosis and management of acute heart failure. In: Gaggin HK, Januzzi JL. *MGH cardiology board review.* London: Springer London; 2013:238–254. (doi: 10.1007/978-1-4471-4483-0)

7. Matsue Y, Damman K, Voors AA, et al. Time-to-furosemide treatment and mortality in patients hospitalized with acute heart failure. *J Am Coll Cardiol.* 2017;69:3042–3051. (doi: 10.1016/j.jacc.2017.04.042)

CHAPTER 4

CHRONIC CHF

NYHA CLASSIFICATION

I – No symptoms with ordinary activity

II – Symptoms with ordinary physical activity

III – Symptoms with less than ordinary physical activity

IV – Rest symptoms and/or inability to carry out any physical activity without symptoms

ACC/AHA CLASSIFICATION

- ○ A – High risk for developing CHF
  - ● HTN, DM, CAD, FH cardiomyopathy
- ○ B – Asymptomatic structural heart disease
  - ● MI, Valve disease, asymptomatic LV dysfunction
- ○ C – Symptomatic heart failure
  - ● NYHA Class II–III
- ○ D – Refractory end stage heart failure
  - ● Symptoms at rest despite max therapy

STANDARD MEDICAL THERAPY FOR CHF WITH REDUCED EF (≤ 40%)

- Beta-blocker
  - Carvedilol, metoprolol succinate, bisoprolol
- ACE/ARB
- Nitrates/hydralazine
  - Indicated in African American patients with persistent Class III–IV symptoms despite treatment with ACE/ARB and beta-blocker
  - Can also be used in place of ACE/ARB in patients who cannot tolerate or have contraindication to ACE/ARB
- Aldosterone antagonist
  - Spironolactone / eplerenone
  - Indicated for persistent Class II–IV symptoms in patients already receiving ACE/ARB and beta-blocker / or asymptomatic patients with DM (also on ACE/ARB/BB)
  - Contraindicated if potassium > 5 / creatinine > 2.0 in females or > 2.5 in males
- Diuretic
  - Relieve congestion / symptoms of SOB
  - No proven mortality benefit
- Echocardiogram is indicated to evaluate EF anytime there is a significant change in clinical status or 3–6 months after optimizing medical therapy

HEART FAILURE WITH PRESERVED EJECTION FRACTION

- E – Peak velocity of early left ventricular filling
- A – Peak velocity of late left ventricular filling
- e' – Peak tissue Doppler velocity of the tissue adjacent to the mitral valve annulus
- Normal values
  - E/A > 1.0 and < 2.0
  - Septal e' ≥ 8 cm/s
  - Lateral e' ≥ 10 cm/s
  - LA volume < 34 mL/m^2
- Diastolic dysfunction – echocardiographic findings
- Impaired LV relaxation with normal filling pressures (grade I diastolic dysfunction)
  - Prolonged deceleration time > 220 ms
  - E/A ratio < 1
  - E < 50 cm/s
  - Septal / lateral e' / LA volume all normal
- Elevated LA pressure (grade II / III diastolic dysfunction)
  - E/A ≥ 2
  - Deceleration time < 200 ms
  - E/e' > 14
  - Septal e' < 8 cm/s
  - Lateral e' < 10 cm/s
  - LA volume index > 34 mL/m^2

- Treated similar to heart failure with reduced ejection fraction
  - Diuretics to decrease congestion is the mainstay of treatment
- No treatments **proven** to prolong survival or decrease hospitalizations

DEVICE THERAPY

- CRT
  - Only indicated after 3 months of goal directed medical therapy
  - Indications
    - EF ≤ 35%, NYHA Class II – ambulatory Class IV despite maximal medical therapy **AND** QRS > 120 ms **AND** LBBB morphology (strongest evidence for QRS > 150 ms)
- ICD
  - Indications
    - EF ≤ 35%, NYHA Class II–III despite maximal medical therapy
    - EF < 30%, NYHA Class I
    - Both indications require patient to be > 40 days post-MI or > 90 days post-revascularization or > 90 days of goal directed medical therapy in NICM
- Combining an ICD with CRT based upon the indications for ICD therapy

MECHANICAL CIRCULATORY SUPPORT

○ Impella
  ◉ Cannula across aortic valve into LV; blood ejected from LV to ascending aorta

○ TandemHeart
  ◉ Left atrium to femoral artery bypass

○ Extracorporeal membrane oxygenation
  ◉ Supports both left and right heart

○ All require systemic anticoagulation

TRANSPLANT

○ Indications
  ◉ Inotrope dependence
  ◉ Refractory, non-revascularizable angina
  ◉ Refractory ventricular arrhythmias
  ◉ Unresectable myocardial tumors without metastases

○ Cardiopulmonary exercise testing (should not be used as lone criteria for transplant)
  ◉ Peak VO_2 < 14 mL/kg/min (< 12 if on BB)
  ◉ Peak VO_2 < 50% predicted

- Transplant contraindications
  - Severe PVD
  - Active infection
  - Severe cerebral vascular disease
  - Noncompliance / poor social support
  - Pulmonary hypertension
    - PA pressure > 60 mmHg / pulmonary vascular resistance > 5 WU / transpulmonary gradient > 15
    - May still be listed if pulmonary pressures can be lowered with vasodilator or mechanical support (IABP/LVAD)
  - Age > 70
  - Malignancy
  - BMI > 30
  - Tobacco / Drugs
    - Typically require 6 months of abstinence before being listed

- Transplant complications
  - Rejection → Diagnosed by endomyocardial biopsy
    - Hyperacute rejection (minutes to hours)
      - Due to preformed ABs
    - Acute cellular rejection (1 week to 6 months)
      - T-cell mediated / treat with pulsed dose steroids
    - Humoral rejection
      - Antibody-mediated / treat with enhanced immunosuppression or AB-depleting therapies

- Cardiac allograft vasculopathy
  - Progressive intimal thickening of the coronaries
    - Diagnosed by IVUS
    - Treat with statins (pravastatin) / no role for PCI / often requires re-transplant for definitive treatment
- Malignancy
  - Most common cause of death > 5 years post-transplant
  - B-cell lymphoma most common secondary to Epstein-Barr virus infection

REFERENCES

1. The Criteria Committee of the New York Heart Association. *Nomenclature and criteria for diagnosis of diseases of the heart and great vessels.* 9th ed. Little, Brown & Co, Boston;1994:253–256.

2. Yancy CW, Jessup M, Bozkurt B, et al. 2013 ACCF/AHA guideline for the management of heart failure: A report of the American College of Cardiology Foundation/American Heart Association Task Force on Practice Guidelines. *J Am Coll Cardiol.* 2013;62:e147–239. (doi: 10.1016/j.jacc.2013.05.019)

3. Yancy CW, Jessup M, Bozkurt B, et al. 2017 ACC/AHA/HFSA focused update of the 2013 ACCF/AHA guideline for the management of heart failure: A report of the American College of Cardiology/American Heart Association Task Force on Clinical Practice Guidelines and the Heart Failure Society of America. *J Am Coll Cardiol.* 2017;70:776–803. (doi: 10.1016/j.jacc.2017.04.025)

4. Nagueh SF, Otto A. Smiseth OA, Christopher P. Appleton CP, et al. Recommendations for the Evaluation of Left Ventricular Diastolic Function by Echocardiography: An update from the American Society of Echocardiography and the European Association of Cardiovascular Imaging. *J Am Soc Echocardiogr.* 2016;29:277–314. (doi: 10.1016/j.echo.2016.01.011)

5. Tracy CM, Epstein AE, Darbar D, et al. 2012 ACCF/AHA/HRS focused update of the 2008 guidelines for device-based therapy of cardiac rhythm abnormalities. *J Am Coll Cardiol.* 2012;60(14):1297–1313. (doi: 10.1016/j.jacc.2012.07.009)

6. Yancy CW, Jessup M, Bozkurt B, et al. 2016 ACC/AHA/HFSA Focused Update on New Pharmacological Therapy for Heart Failure: An update of the 2013 ACCF/AHA guideline for the management of heart failure. *J Am Coll Cardiol.* 2016;68:1476–1488. (doi: 10.1016/j.jacc.2016.05.011)

7. Mehra MR, Canter CE, Hannan MM, et al. The 2016 International Society for Heart Lung Transplantation listing criteria for heart transplantation: A 10-year update. *J Heart Lung Transplant.* 2016;35:1–23. (doi: 10.1016/j.healun.2015.10.023)

8. Mehra MR, Kobashigawa J, Starling R, et al. Listing criteria for heart transplantation: International Society for Heart and Lung Transplantation Guidelines for the care of cardiac transplant candidates – 2006. *J Heart Lung Transplant.* 2006;25:1024–1042. (doi: 10.1016/j.healun.2006.06.008)

HYPERTROPHIC CARDIOMYOPATHY

HYPERTROPHIC CARDIOMYOPATHY

○ Diagnosis
  - LVH with septal thickness > 15 mm in the absence of LV pressure overload
  - Septum: posterior wall ratio > 1.3:1

○ Physical exam essentials
  - Double peaked (bisferiens) pulse
  - Murmur heard best at left lower sternal border
    • Murmur increases in intensity with ↓ preload / ↓ afterload / **following PVC**
  - Brockenbrough sign
    • ↓ pulse pressure following PVC due to increased outflow obstruction produced by enhanced contractility of the post-PVC beat
    • Versus aortic stenosis → pulse pressure will not fall post-PVC

- Major risk factors for sudden cardiac death
  - Septum > 30 mm
  - History of syncope
  - Less than 20 mmHg systolic blood pressure increase with exercise
  - Family history of sudden death
  - VT on Holter monitor

- Treatment
  - Negative inotropes / chronotropes to treat symptoms → beta-blockers, non-dihydropyridine calcium-channel blockers
  - No competitive sports
    - Billiards, bowling, cricket, riflery, curling OK
  - Warfarin for **all afib** even with CHADS-VASc score 0–1
  - Myectomy for refractory symptoms
    - Septal ablation only if prohibitive surgical risk
  - ICD indicated in all patients with 1 or more risk factor for sudden cardiac death
  - No indication for PPM unless there is some other indication for pacing

- Family screening
  - Echo / ECG in all first-degree relatives
  - Age 12–18 → echo and ECG every 12–18 months
  - Age > 18 → echo and ECG every 5 years
    - Every 12–18 months if competing in athletics
  - Genetic testing only useful if index patient + for HCM mutation
    - Relatives who are mutation negative do not require screening

REFERENCES

1. Maron BJ. Hypertrophic cardiomyopathy: A systematic review. *JAMA*. 2002;287:1308–1320. (doi: 10.1001/jama.287.10.1308)

2. Gersh BJ, Maron BJ, Bonow RO, et al. 2011 ACCF/AHA guideline for the diagnosis and treatment of hypertrophic cardiomyopathy: executive summary: A report of the American College of Cardiology Foundation/American Heart Association Task Force on Practice Guidelines. *Circulation*. 2011;124:2761–2796. (doi: 10.1161/CIR.0b013e318223e230)

CHAPTER 6

CARDIAC CHANNELOPATHIES

BRUGADA SYNDROME

- Males predominate (4:1)

- Southeast Asian ancestry is most common

- Loss of function in 5CN5A sodium channel

- Role of EP evaluation for diagnosis is unclear

- No indication for ICD for primary prevention / only indicated after aborted sudden cardiac death (SCD)

- Quinidine useful in the setting of repetitive ICD shocks

CATECHOLAMINERGIC POLYMORPHIC VENTRICULAR TACHYCARDIA

- ○ Typically triggered by exercise
- ○ No indication for ICD for primary prevention
  - ● ICD indicated for aborted SCD / always in conjunction with a beta-blocker
- ○ ICD is never the lone treatment → ICD shock can trigger further VT
- ○ Beta-blocker (nadolol) +/– flecainide for treatment when no ICD indication

LONG QT SYNDROME (LQTS)

- ○ No indication for ICD for primary prevention in LQTS (including FH of SCD)
- ○ Normal QTc
  - ● < 450 ms in males
  - ● < 460 ms in females
- ○ Only way to **definitively** exclude channelopathy is a known mutation in a family member and the individual in question testing negative for that mutation
- ○ Long QT 1
  - ● Loss of function in KCNQ1 potassium channel
  - ● Arrhythmia classically exercise triggered
  - ● Treat with beta-blockers

- ○ Long QT 2
  - ● Notched T waves seen on ECG
  - ● Loss of function in KCNQ2 potassium channel
  - ● Arrhythmia triggered by sudden noises / startle
    - • Also manifests more frequently with pregnancy

- ○ Long QT 3
  - ● Long, isoelectric baseline with normal appearing T waves
  - ● Gain of function in 5CN5A sodium channel
  - ● Sudden death during inactivity / sleep

REFERENCE

1. Priori SG, Wilde AA, Horie M, et al. HRS/EHRA/APHRS expert consensus statement on the diagnosis and management of patients with inherited primary arrhythmia syndromes. *Heart Rhythm.* 2013;10:1932–1963. (doi: 10.1016/j.hrthm.2013.05.014)

SUPRAVENTRICULAR ARRHYTHMIAS

ATRIAL FIBRILLATION (AF)

- ○ Paroxysmal atrial fibrillation (PAF)
  - AF that spontaneously converts to NSR in < 7 days
- ○ Persistent atrial fibrillation
  - AF > 7 days' duration or ≥ 48 hours but < 7 days in patient who is cardioverted
- ○ Chronic atrial fibrillation
  - AF > 12 months' duration
- ○ CHADS-VASc score
  - One point each for:
    - CHF (clinical diagnosis or EF < 40%)
    - HTN
    - Age 65–74
      - ○ 2 points for age ≥ 75
    - Diabetes mellitus
    - Vascular disease (prior MI, PAD, aortic plaque)
    - Female sex
  - 2 points for:
    - History of CVA or TIA

○ Approximate stroke risk based on CHADS-VASc score
  ◦ 1–4 → 1%–4% risk respectively
  ◦ 5 → ~7%
  ◦ 6–7 → ~10%
  ◦ 9 → ~15%
○ Anticoagulation
  ◦ As a general rule, in the absence of significant bleeding risk, always anticoagulate if CHADS-VASc ≥ 2
  ◦ Warfarin
    • INR goal 2.0–3.0
  ◦ Novel oral anticoagulants (NOAC)
    • Dabigatran (Pradaxa)
      ○ Direct thrombin inhibitor
      ○ 150 mg PO bid
        ‣ Age > 75 or CrCl 15–30 → 75 mg PO bid
      ○ Contraindicated if creatinine < 15 or hepatic failure
    • Rivaroxaban (Xarelto)
      ○ Xa inhibitor
      ○ 20 mg PO qHS
        ‣ CrCL 15–50 → 15 mg PO qHS
      ○ Contraindicated if creatinine < 15 or hepatic failure
    • Apixaban (Eliquis)
      ○ Xa inhibitor
      ○ 5 mg PO bid
        ‣ Any 2 of the following:
        ‣ Cr > 1.5 mg/dL / age > 80 / weight < 60 kg → 2.5 mg PO bid

- Holding NOACs prior to surgery
  - High bleeding risk → hold 48 hours prior
  - Low bleeding risk → hold 24 hours prior
  - In general, the rapid onset and offset of action of the NOACs eliminates the need for bridging when interrupting anticoagulation

○ Catheter ablation of atrial fibrillation
  - Class I indication for patients with symptomatic atrial fibrillation who have failed or not tolerated at least one antiarrhythmic
    - Chest CT 3 months postablation in all patients to exclude pulmonary vein stenosis
  - Atrial-esophageal fistula is the most feared complication
    - Typically occurs 1–4 weeks postablation
    - Presents with sepsis / CNS symptoms
      ○ Surgical emergency
      ○ **Do not** perform endoscopy due to high risk of rupture

○ Antiarrhythmics
  - See Chapter 29: Pharmacology Essentials

ATRIAL FLUTTER

○ Indications for anticoagulation and anticoagulant options are identical to atrial fibrillation

○ Adenosine / vagal maneuvers can be used to unmask atrial flutter waves but does not typically terminate the arrhythmia, since the AV node is not involved in the circuit

- Atrial flutter ablation
  - Typical (counterclockwise) flutter is often cured by radiofrequency ablation of the **cavotricuspid isthmus**
    - No formal guideline recommendations governing atrial flutter ablation
  - Atypical (clockwise) flutter is less reliably cured by ablation

- Rate vs. rhythm control
  - Rhythm control strategy does not reduce stroke risk or alter the need for anticoagulation
  - Once afib/flutter diagnosed, decision for anticoagulation should be based on CHADS-VASc score, regardless of rhythm at the current time
  - Cardioversion within 48 hours of arrhythmia onset → patients at high risk for stroke should be treated with a NOAC, LMWH, or UFH, before or immediately following cardioversion and subsequently started on long term oral anticoagulation (Ic recommendation)
  - Afib/flutter > 48 hours or unknown duration → requires therapeutic anticoagulation 3 weeks prior to cardioversion and a minimum of 4 weeks after
    - TEE to exclude intracardiac thrombus can be performed in lieu of 3 weeks of anticoagulation prior
      - Does not change the need for anticoagulation following cardioversion

AV NODAL REENTRANT TACHYCARDIA (AVNRT)

○ Requires dual AV node physiology with differing conduction velocities
  - Rapid conduction velocity → longer refractory period
  - Slow conduction velocity → shorter refractory period
  - This variation creates a period where one pathway is refractory while the other has recovered and is able to conduct
    - An appropriately timed atrial premature contraction will conduct over one pathway but block in the pathway still in its refractory period
    - If the previously blocked pathway has recovered by the time conduction over the first pathway is complete, the impulse can enter the previously refractory pathway in a retrograde fashion and set up a reciprocating tachycardia

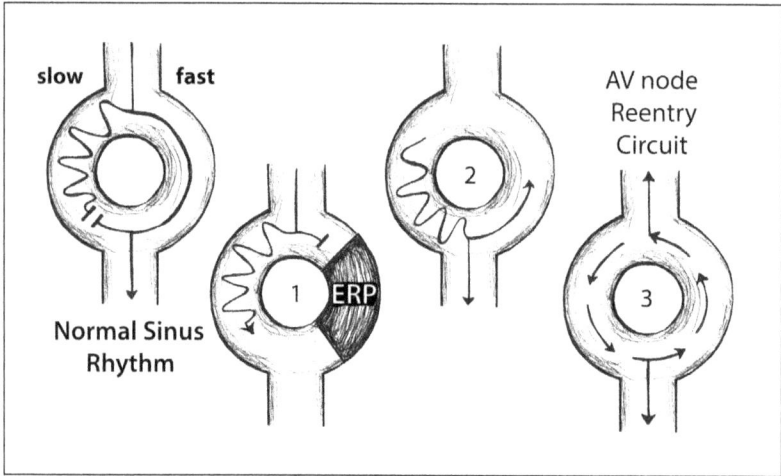

Figure 7.1 AVNRT.
(1) An atrial premature contraction is able to conduct antegrade over the slow pathway but is blocked in the still refractory fast pathway; (2) By the time conduction over the slow pathway is complete, the fast pathway has recovered and is no longer refractory, allowing retrograde conduction "up" the fast pathway; (3) By the time the impulse has conducted retrograde over the fast pathway, the slow pathway has recovered and is again able to conduct the impulse in the antegrade direction, creating a reentrant circuit (typical slow-fast AVNRT).

- ○ Typical slow-fast AVNRT
  - ◉ Antegrade conduction conduction via the slow pathway with retrograde conduction via the fast pathway
    - ECG → rapid, narrow complex tachycardia with pseudo R′ in V_1 and V_2 and pseudo S waves in the inferior leads (due to retrograde conduction back to the ventricle)
  - ◉ Treatment
    - Vagal maneuvers / carotid massage
    - Adenosine 6 mg or 12 mg rapid IV push
      - ○ Leads to block in the AV node and termination of the arrhythmia
    - Ablation of the slow pathway is most effective definitive treatment

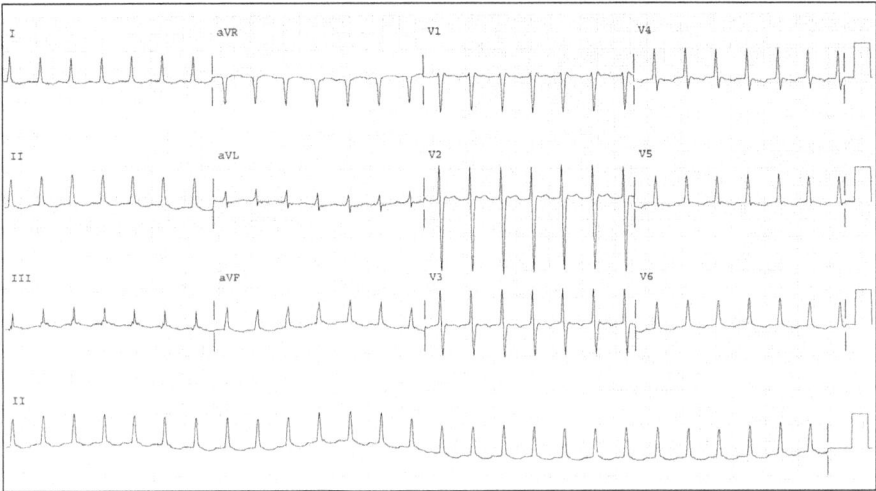

Figure 7.2 Typical AVNRT.
Reprinted with permission. AVNRT for two. September 30, 2009 by Mike Cadogan.
https://lifeinthefastlane.com/avnrtecg/

AV REENTRANT TACHYCARDIA (AVRT)

- Mechanism of initiation and maintenance of the arrhythmia is identical to AVNRT
  - Difference is the entire circuit does not reside within the AV node
- Wolff-Parkinson-White is most common type of AVRT
- Orthodromic AVRT → Antegrade conduction via the AV node with retrograde conduction via the bypass tract
  - Narrow complex tachycardia
- Antidromic AVRT → antegrade conduction over the bypass tract with retrograde conduction via the AV node
  - Wide complex / short R-P tachycardia

- ○ "Concealed" accessory pathway → conducts only in retrograde fashion
  - Concealed because there is no delta wave on the ECG

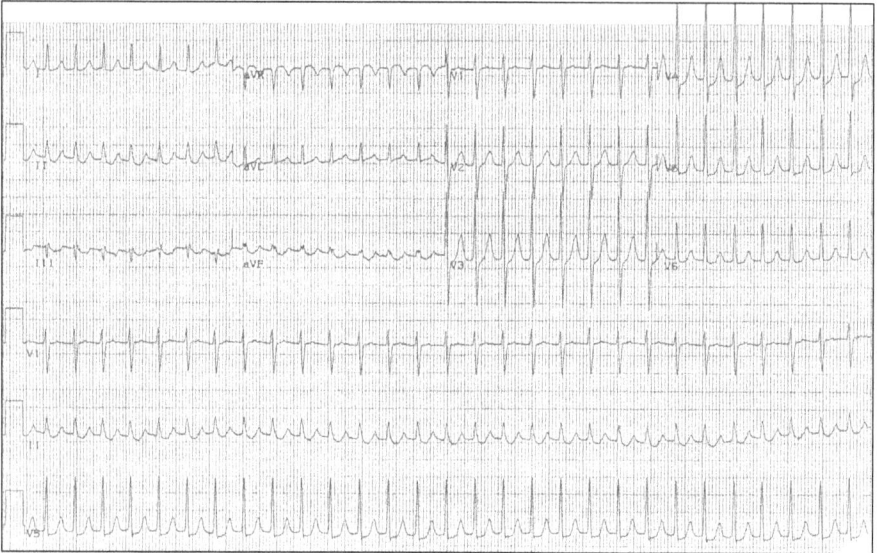

Figure 7.3 Orthodromic AVRT.
Reprinted with permission. Life in the Fast Lane. Preexcitation Syndromes.
https://lifeinthefastlane.com/ecglibrary/preexcitationsyndromes/

AFIB AND WPW

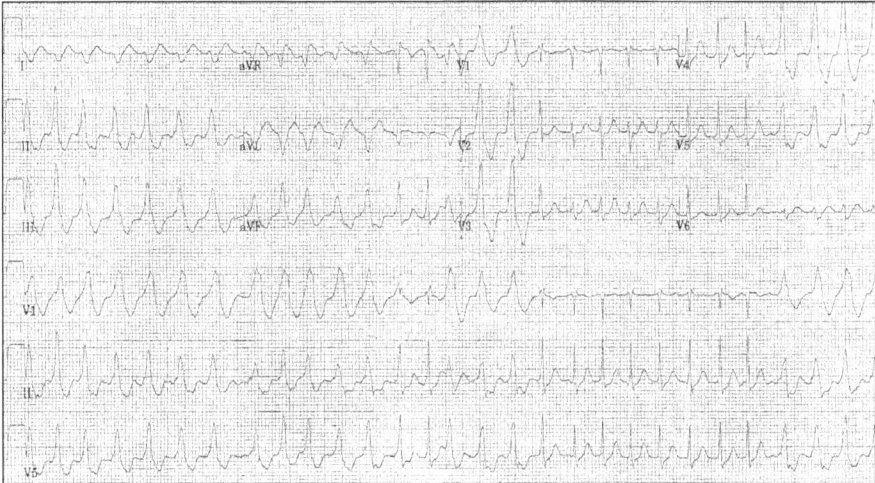

Figure 7.4 Afib with WPW.
Reprinted with permission. Life in the Fast Lane. Preexcitation Syndromes.
https://lifeinthefastlane.com/ecglibrary/preexcitationsyndromes/

○ Treatment options:
- Cardioversion
- Amiodarone or procainamide
- **Never use calcium channel blockers, beta-blockers, or adenosine**
  - Can slow conduction through the AV node → preferential conduction over the bypass tract → hemodynamic collapse
- Digoxin contraindicated in patients with preexcitation
  - Shortens the refractory period of the accessory pathway

REFERENCES

1. January CT, Wann LS, Alpert JS, et al. 2014 AHA/ACC/HRS guide-line for the management of patients with atrial fibrillation: A report of the American College of Cardiology/American Heart Association Task Force on Practice Guidelines and the Heart Rhythm Society. *Circulation.* 2014;130:e199–e267.

2. Page RL, Joglar JA, Caldwell MA, et al. 2015 ACC/AHA/HRS guideline for the management of adult patients with supraventricular tachycardia: A report of the American College of Cardiology/American Heart Association Task Force on Clinical Practice Guidelines and the Heart Rhythm Society. *Circulation.* 2016;133:e506–e574.

CHAPTER 8

VENTRICULAR ARRHYTHMIAS AND DEFIBRILLATORS

CLASS I INDICATIONS FOR ICD IMPLANTATION

- ○ Cardiac arrest due to VT/VF without a reversible cause (**≥ 48 hours post-MI**)

- ○ Sustained VT in the setting of structural heart disease

- ○ Syncope of unknown cause with inducible VT/VF at EPS

- ○ LVEF ≤ 35% due to MI ≥ 40 days prior with Class II or III symptoms
  - If revascularized following MI, need to reassess EF 90 days following MI to determine candidacy for ICD

- ○ Nonischemic cardiomyopathy, EF ≤ 35%, Class II or III symptoms, after at least 3 months of medical therapy

- ○ Prior MI with **Class I** symptoms and EF ≤ 30%

- ○ Prior MI, LVEF ≤ 40%, nonsustained VT, inducible at EPS

CLASS III

○ Survival < 1 year

○ Incessant VT/VF

○ Refractory, Class IV symptoms in someone who is not a transplant or CRT candidate

RIGHT VENTRICULAR OUTFLOW TRACT TACHYCARDIA

○ Typically benign and usually responds to beta-blockers, calcium-channel blockers, or ablation

○ 10% PVC burden increases the risk for cardiomyopathy → typically treat with ablation

○ ECG → LBBB morphology / inferior axis

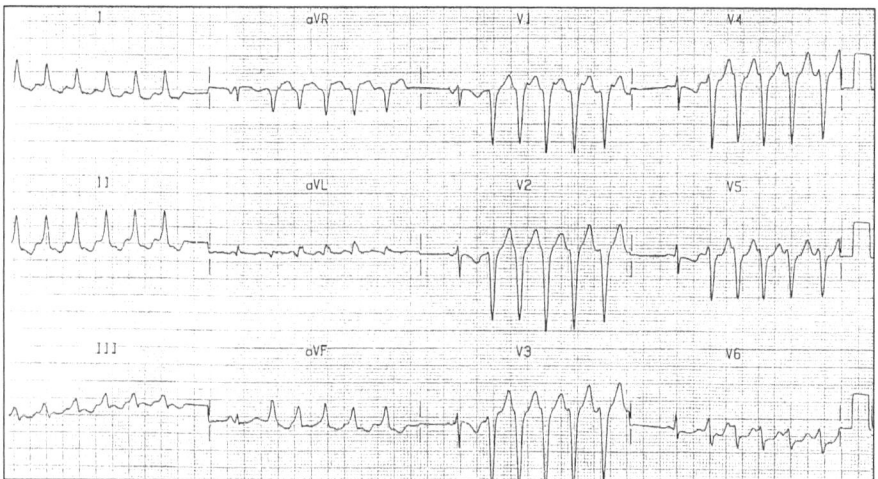

Figure 8.1 RVOT VT.
Used with permission from Podrid P, Malhotra R, Kakar R, Noseworthy PA. *Podrid's Real-World ECGs: A Master's Approach to the Art and Practice of Clinical ECG Interpretation, Volume 4A*. Minneapolis, MN: Cardiotext Publishing; 2015.

FASCICULAR VT

○ ECG → RBBB morphology / superior axis

○ Responds to verapamil

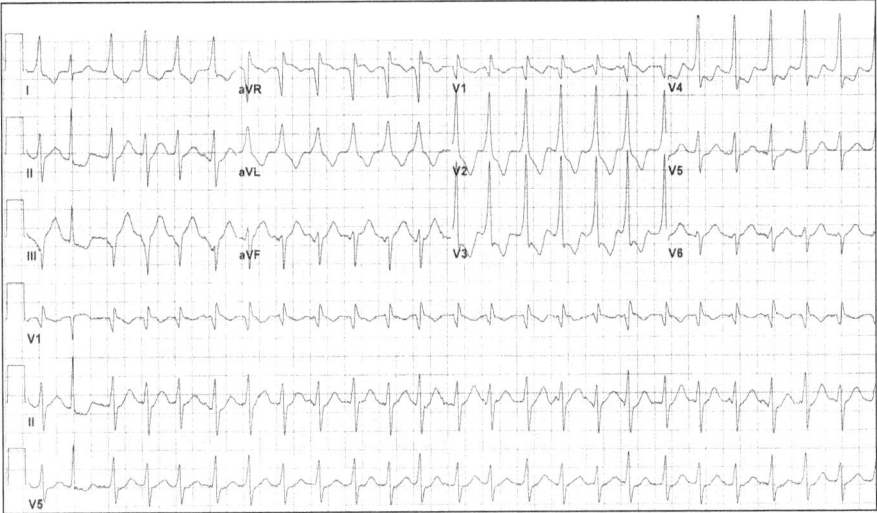

Figure 8.2 Fascicular VT.
Used with permission from Podrid P, Malhotra R, Kakar R, Noseworthy PA. *Podrid's Real-World ECGs: A Master's Approach to the Art and Practice of Clinical ECG Interpretation, Volume 5A*. Minneapolis, MN: Cardiotext Publishing; 2016.

ARRHYTHMOGENIC RIGHT VENTRICULAR DYSPLASIA

ECG → QRS widening / T-wave inversions V_1–V_3 / abnormal terminal portion of the QRS (epsilon wave)

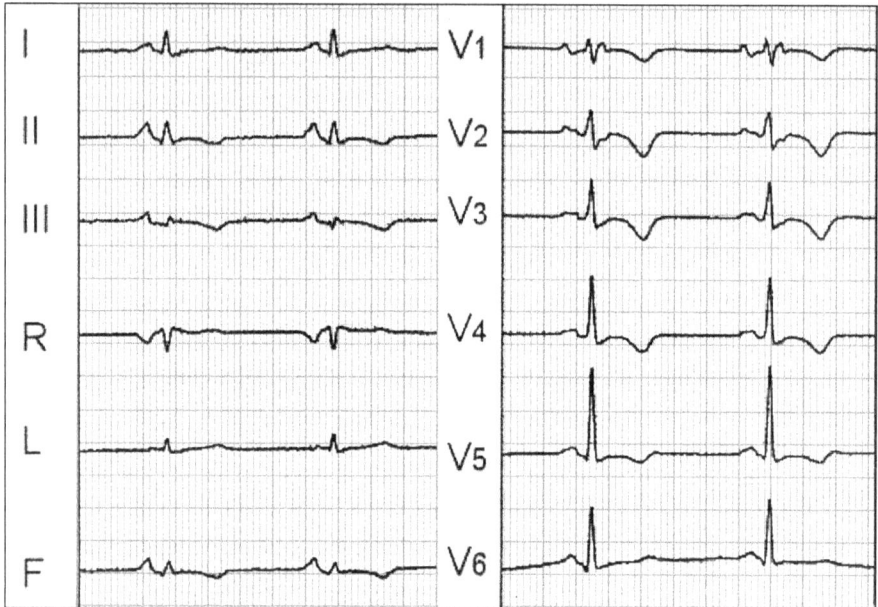

Figure 8.3 Arrhythmogenic right ventricular dysplasia.
Used with permission from Podrid P, Malhotra R, Kakar R, Noseworthy PA. *Podrid's Real-World ECGs: A Master's Approach to the Art and Practice of Clinical ECG Interpretation, Volume 6.* Minneapolis, MN: Cardiotext Publishing; 2016.

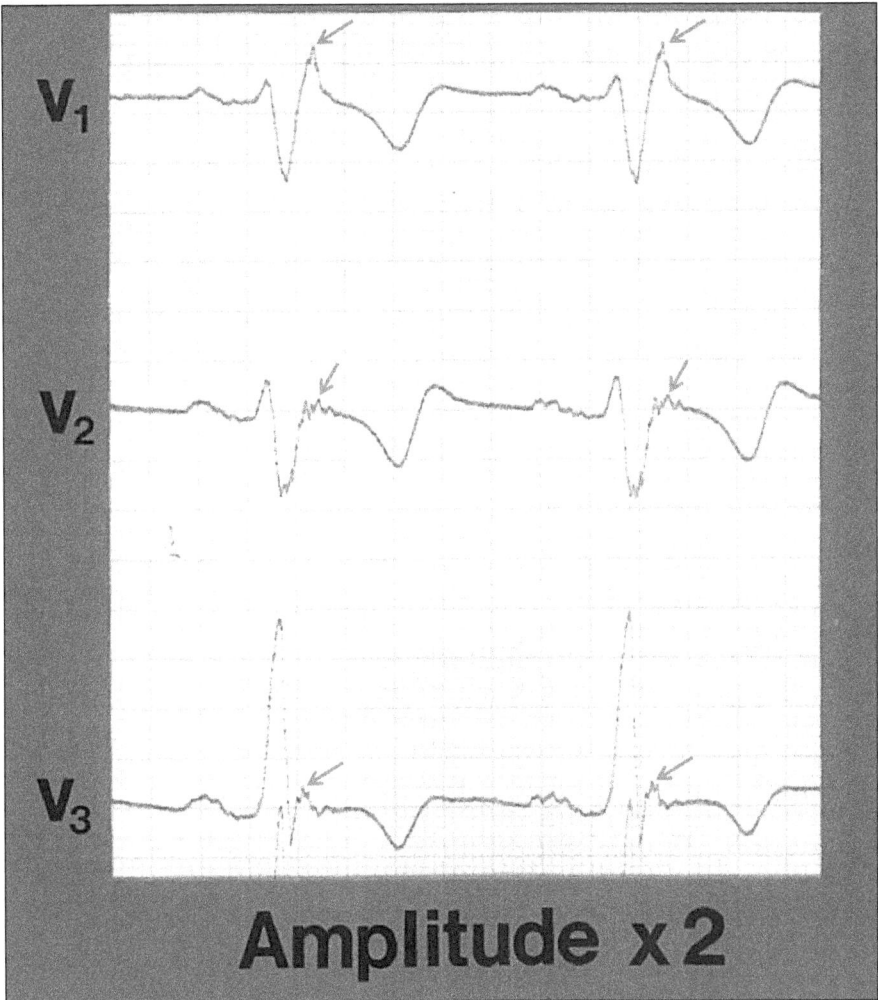

Figure 8.4 Arrhythmogenic right ventricular dysplasia. Arrow indicates epsilon wave. Cardiac MRI typically part of the diagnostic workup.

Used with permission from Podrid P, Malhotra R, Kakar R, Noseworthy PA. *Podrid's Real-World ECGs: A Master's Approach to the Art and Practice of Clinical ECG Interpretation, Volume 5A*. Minneapolis, MN: Cardiotext Publishing; 2016.

REFERENCES

1. Tracy CM, Epstein AE, Darbar D, et al. 2012 ACCF/AHA/HRS focused update of the 2008 guidelines for device-based therapy of cardiac rhythm abnormalities. *J Am Coll Cardiol.* 2012;60(14):1297–1313. (doi: 10.1016/j.jacc.2012.07.009)

2. Yancy CW, Jessup M, Bozkurt B, et al. 2013 ACCF/AHA guideline for the management of heart failure: A report of the American College of Cardiology Foundation/American Heart Association Task Force on Practice Guidelines. *J Am Coll Cardiol.* 2013;62:e147–239. (doi: 10.1016/j.jacc.2013.05.019)

CHAPTER 9

BRADYCARDIA / PACEMAKERS

- ○ Sinus arrhythmia
  - ● INspiration INhibits vagal tone → INcreased HR
  - ● HR decreases with expiration

- ○ Carotid sinus hypersensitivity
  - ● Profound sinus bradycardia / pauses from pressure on the carotids
  - ● Recurrent syncope with evidence that carotid pressure produces pauses > 3 seconds → Class I indication for PPM

- ○ Sinus node dysfunction
  - ● Class I indications for PPM
  - ● Documented symptomatic bradycardia / pauses
  - ● Symptomatic chronotropic incompetence
  - ● Symptomatic bradycardia from required drug therapy

- SA exit block
  - First-degree cannot be seen on surface ECG
  - Second-degree type I → progressive shortening of P-P interval until P wave dropped
  - Second-degree type II → sinus pause is **exact** multiple of preceding R-R interval
  - Third-degree → sinus arrest
- AV block
  - Mobitz I → progressive P-R prolongation / progressive shortening of R-R interval until dropped QRS
    - Block within AV node
    - Typically followed clinically / does not require PPM
  - Mobitz II → Sudden nonconduction of atrial impulse without change in preceding P-R interval
    - Infranodal block
    - Requires PPM

PACEMAKERS

- Nomenclature
  - Paced / sensed / response (to sensed event) / Rate modulation
  - First letter describes pacing location
    - A → Atrium paces
    - V → Ventricle paces
    - D → Dual / both chambers pace
    - O → Neither
  - Second letter describes chamber sensed with same code as above

- Third letter describes response to sensing
  - I → Inhibit pacing
  - T → Trigger pacing
  - D → Inhibit and / or trigger pacing (i.e., sensed event in atrium will lead to triggered pacing in the ventricle after a programmable time period if no sensed event occurs in the ventricle, which would inhibit pacing)
  - O → No response
- Fourth letter describes the presence or absence of rate modulation
  - R → Rate response active
  - O → No rate response
- Example, VVIR
  - Ventricular paced / ventricular sensed / Inhibit pacing / rate response active
- Hysteresis
  - Device occasionally allows V rate below set limit in order to facilitate intrinsic conduction
  - Often confused with oversensing
- VVIR → used frequently in chronic afib
  - Can lead to pacemaker syndrome
    - Atrial contraction against closed MV / TV → decreased stroke volume, sense of dizziness / weakness
  - Basic rule: No need for atrial lead in chronic afib/flutter
  - Dual chamber device in all others

- Most common Class I indications for PPM
  - Third-degree AV block + symptoms
  - Third-degree AV block / no symptoms / **AND**:
    - Asystole ≥ 3.0 seconds
    - Escape rate < 40 bpm
    - Escape rhythm below AV node
    - Post-op, not expected to improve
    - ANY neuromuscular disease
  - Afib with pauses > 5 seconds
  - Second- or third-degree AV block during exercise
  - Mobitz II
  - Alternating bundle branch block
  - Carotid sinus hypersensitivity
    - Symptomatic pauses ≥ 3.0 seconds
    - Asymptomatic ≥ 6 seconds (2A indication)

REFERENCES

1. Epstein AE, DiMarco JP, Ellenbogen KA, et al. ACC/AHA/HRS 2008 guidelines for device-based therapy of cardiac rhythm abnormalities: Executive summary: A report of the American College of Cardiology/American Heart Association Task Force on Practice Guidelines (Writing Committee to Revise the ACC/AHA/NASPE 2002 Guideline Update for Implantation of Cardiac Pacemakers and Antiarrhythmia Devices). *J Am Coll Cardiol.* 2008;51:2085–105. (doi:10.1016/j.jacc.2008.02.033)

2. Hesselson AB. Chapter 9: The code and mode. In: Hesselson AB. *Simplified interpretation of pacemaker ECGs.* New York: Blackwell Publishing / Futura; 2003:65–70.

CHAPTER 10

VALVULAR HEART DISEASE

AORTIC STENOSIS

- ○ Physical exam essentials
  - ◉ Reduced carotid upstrokes
  - ◉ Diminished A2
  - ◉ Mid to late peaking murmur
    - • Later peaking = more severe
  - ◉ Ejection sound / click indicative of bicuspid valve
  - ◉ Murmur ↑ with ↑ preload / ↓ with ↑ afterload

Table 10.1 Grading Severity of Aortic Stenosis

	Mild	Severe
Peak gradient	< 3.0 m/s	> 4.0 m/s
Mean gradient	< 20 mmHg	> 40 mmHg
Aortic valve area	> 1.5 cm²	< 1.0 cm²
Indexed aortic valve area	> 0.85 cm²/m²	< 0.6 cm²/m²
Velocity ratio/ dimensionless index	> 0.5	< 0.25

- ○ Natural history (50% survival)
  - Angina → 5 years
  - Syncope → 3 years
  - CHF → 2 years
- ○ Follow-up
  - Mild AS → repeat echo in 3–5 years
  - Moderate AS → repeat echo in 1–2 years
  - Severe AS → repeat echo every 6–12 months
- ○ Surgical indications
  - Severe AS + symptoms
  - Severe AS / undergoing other cardiac surgery (moderate AS = IIB indication)
  - Severe AS / asymptomatic AND EF < 50%

AORTIC INSUFFICIENCY

- ○ Physical exam essentials
  - Waterhammer pulse / wide pulse pressure
  - Murmur heard best at left sternal border / sitting up / leaning forward / end expiration
  - **Acute**, severe AI → short, early diastolic murmur (due to rapid equalization of pressures), diastolic MR

Table 10.2 Grading Severity of Aortic Insufficiency

	Mild	Severe
Jet width/LVOT	< 0.25	> 0.65
Vena contracta	< 0.3 cm	> 0.6 cm
Pressure half time	> 500 ms	< 200 ms
Regurgitant volume	< 30 mL/beat	> 60 mL/beat
Regurgitant fraction	< 30%	> 50%
Regurgitant orifice area	< 0.1 cm²	> 0.3 cm²

- Acute management
  - Vasodilators for acute, severe AI to reduce afterload
    - **Nitroprusside**, hydralazine
- Follow-up
  - Mild AI → repeat echo in 3–5 years
  - Moderate AI → repeat echo every 1–2 years
  - Severe AI → repeat echo every 6–12 months
- Surgical indications
  - Severe AI + symptoms
  - Severe AI / Asymptomatic **AND** any one of the following:
    - EF < 50%
    - Other cardiac surgery
    - End diastolic dimension > 65 mm or end systolic dimension > 50 mm

MITRAL STENOSIS

- Normal transmitral diastolic velocity < 1.3 m/s
- Rheumatic fever is most common cause of mitral stenosis
- Symptoms primarily related to ↑ LA pressure → transmitted to the pulmonary vasculature
- Patients tend to tolerate tachycardia poorly
  - ↓ diastolic filling time → ↑ LA pressures
- Physical exam essentials
  - Loud S1
  - Opening snap
    - S2/OS interval decreases with increasing MS severity
  - Mid-diastolic murmur

○ Calculations to know
  ● Mitral valve area = 220/pressure half time (PHT)
    • PHT = Vmax/1.4
    • PHT = deceleration time × 0.29

Table 10.3 Grading Severity of Mitral Stenosis

	Mild	Severe
Mean gradient	< 5 mmHg	> 10 mmHg
Mitral valve area	> 1.5 cm²	< 1.0 cm²
PA systolic pressure	< 30 mmHg	> 50 mmHg

○ **Balloon valvuloplasty preferred over MV surgery in patients without contraindications**
  ● Contraindications to mitral balloon valvuloplasty
    • Wilkins score > 8
    • Moderate or severe MR
    • LA thrombus
○ Wilkins score
  ● Each of the four components of the Wilkins score is given a grade of 1 to 4 relative to increasing severity
  ● Only grades 1 and 4 are listed in Table 10.4, as it is not necessary to memorize each grade

Table 10.4 Wilkins Score

Grade	Leaflet Mobility	Valve Thickening	Subvalvular Disease	Valve Calcification
1	Only the leaflet tips are restricted	4–5 mm	Thickening of chordal structures immediately below the valve	Single, focal area of calcification
4	No / minimal movement of the leaflets	8–10 mm	Thickening and shortening or all chordal structures extending to papillary muscle	Extensive calcification throughout most of leaflet

○ Follow-up
  ◉ MVA > 1.5 cm^2 → repeat echo 3–5 years
  ◉ MVA 1.0–1.5 cm^2 → repeat echo every 1–2 years
  ◉ MVA < 1.0 cm^2 → repeat echo yearly

○ Indications for intervention (valvuloplasty or MVR)
  ◉ **Moderate** or Severe MS + symptoms (**new onset afib considered a symptom**)
  ◉ PASP > 60 mmHg with exercise and/or > 50 mmHg at rest

MITRAL REGURGITATION

○ LA / LV dilate over time → allows accommodation of regurgitant volume at lower pressures → less symptoms

○ EF will be > 60% in compensated MR; any EF < 60% considered abnormal in MR

○ Exam essentials
  ● High pitched, blowing, holosystolic murmur heard best at the apex
  ● Mid-systolic click heard in mitral valve prolapse

Table 10.5 Grading Severity of Mitral Regurgitation

	Mild	Severe
Color jet	Fills < 20% of LA	Fills > 40% of LA
Vena contracta	< 0.3 cm	> 0.7 cm
Regurgitant volume	< 30 mL/beat	> 60 mL/beat
Regurgitant fraction	< 30%	> 50%
Regurgitant orifice area	< 0.2 cm^2	> 0.4 cm^2

○ Follow-up
  ● Mild MR → repeat echo in 3–5 years
  ● Moderate MR → repeat echo 1–2 years
  ● Severe MR → repeat echo every 6–12 months

- ○ Surgical indications (repair **always** favored over replacement when feasible)
  - ● Severe MR + symptoms
  - ● Severe MR / asymptomatic AND
    - • EF < 60% or end systolic dimension ≥ 40 mm
  - ● IIa indications for intervention
    - • Severe / asymptomatic AND any of the following:
      - ○ Likelihood of **repair** > 90%
      - ○ New onset afib
      - ○ PAP > 60 mmHg with exercise and/or 50 mmHg at rest
  - ● Surgical risk significantly increased when EF < 30%

TRICUSPID STENOSIS

- ○ Typically secondary to rheumatic heart disease and coexists with mitral stenosis
- ○ Severe tricuspid stenosis
  - ● Mean gradient > 5 mmHg
  - ● Peak velocity > 2 m/s
  - ● Valve area < 1.0 cm^2
  - ● PHT > 190 ms
- ○ Surgical correction of tricuspid stenosis usually only performed in conjunction with left-sided valve surgery and timing is dictated by severity of the left-sided lesions

TRICUSPID REGURGITATION

- Severe tricuspid regurgitation
  - Regurgitant jet area > 10 cm^2
  - Vena contracta > 0.7 cm
  - Hepatic vein systolic flow reversal

- Only Class I indication for tricuspid repair / replacement is severe TR in patients undergoing MV surgery

PULMONIC STENOSIS

- Carcinoid = most common noncongenital cause

- Physical exam essentials
  - Systolic murmur over left sternal border → radiates to left carotid / increases with inspiration
  - Pulmonic ejection sound
  - Widely split S2 / decreased P2 intensity

- Treatment
  - Balloon valvuloplasty is treatment of choice (Carcinoid may require replacement)

- Indications
  - Symptomatic with mean gradient > 30 mmHg or peak gradient > 50 mmHg
  - Asymptomatic with mean gradient > 50 mmHg

- No consensus guidelines for pulmonic regurgitation

MECHANICAL PROSTHETIC VALVE ANTICOAGULATION

- ○ Aortic position with no risk factors for stroke (afib, prior CVA, EF < 30%, hypercoagulable state), INR goal 2.0–3.0
  - ● Any stroke risk factor → INR 2.5–3.5
- ○ Mechanical mitral prosthesis, goal INR 2.5–3.5
- ○ Anticoagulation prior to noncardiac surgery
  - ● Aortic position, no risk factors → continue ASA only, no bridging
  - ● All others → hold warfarin 5 days pre-op, start LMWH 3 days pre-op, continue ASA throughout

BIOPROSTHETIC VALVE ANTICOAGULATION

- ○ Warfarin (INR goal 2.0–3.0) × 3 months post-op (IIa) + ASA 81 mg daily for life
- ○ TAVR → warfarin (INR goal 2.0–3.0) for 3 months (IIb) or clopidogrel 75 mg daily × 3–6 months (IIb), ASA 81 mg daily for life

REFERENCES

1. Nishimura RA, Otto CM, Bonow RO, et al. 2014 AHA/ACC guide-line for the management of patients with valvular heart disease: A report of the American College of Cardiology/American Heart Association Task Force on Practice Guidelines. *Circulation*. 2014;129:e521–643. (doi: 10.1161/CIR.0000000000000031)

2. Nishimura RA, Otto CM, Bonow RO, et al. 2017 AHA/ACC focused update of the 2014 AHA/ACC guideline for the management of patients with valvular heart disease: A report of the American College of Cardiology/American Heart Association Task Force on Clinical Practice Guidelines. *Circulation*. 2017;135:e1159–1195. (doi: 10.1161/CIR.0000000000000503)

3. Elmariah S, Januzzi JL, Flynn AW, et al. Chapter 16: Valvular heart disease. In: Gaggin HK, Januzzi JL. *MGH cardiology board review.* London: Springer London; 2013:271–297.
(doi: 10.1007/978-1-4471-4483-0)

4. Krishnaswamy A, Griffin BP. Chapter 33: Aortic and pulmonary valve disease. In: Griffin BP, Kapadia SR, Rimmerman CM. *The Cleveland clinic cardiology board review.* 2nd ed. Philadelphia: Lippincott Williams & Wilkins; 2013:461–476.

5. Stewart WJ. Chapter 34: Mitral and tricuspid valve disease. In: Griffin BP, Kapadia SR, Rimmerman CM. *The Cleveland clinic cardiology board review.* 2nd ed. Philadelphia: Lippincott Williams & Wilkins; 2013:477–504.

6. Munt B, Legget ME, Kraft CD, et al. Physical examination in valvular aortic stenosis: Correlation with stenosis severity and prediction of clinical outcome. *Am Heart J.* 1999;137(2):298–306.
(doi: 10.1053/hj.1999.v137.95496)

ENDOCARDITIS

DIAGNOSIS OF ENDOCARDITIS

○ Definite endocarditis (any of the following)
  - Pathology from vegetation
  - 2 major criteria
  - 1 major / 3 minor criteria
  - 5 minor criteria

○ Possible endocarditis (either of the following)
  - 1 major / 1 minor criteria
  - 3 minor criteria

○ Major criteria
  - 2 separate positive blood cultures
    - Single positive blood culture for *Coxiella burnetii*
  - Vegetation on echo
  - Abscess
  - New prosthetic valve dehiscence
  - New valvular regurgitation

- ○ Minor criteria
  - ● Predisposing condition (IVDU)
  - ● Fever > 38°C
  - ● Vascular phenomenon
    - • Emboli / mycotic aneurysms / intracranial hemorrhage / conjunctival hemorrhage / Janeway lesions
- ○ Immunologic phenomena
  - ● Glomerulonephritis / Osler nodes / Roth spots / rheumatoid factor

CLASS I SURGICAL INDICATIONS

- ○ Heart failure
- ○ Valve dehiscence
- ○ Perivalvular abscess
- ○ Fungal endocarditis
- ○ Drug-resistant bacteria
- ○ Persistently positive blood cultures after 1 week of antibiotics
- ○ Embolic events during treatment
- ○ Involvement of anterior MV leaflet (especially if vegetation > 10 mm) → IIa

ENDOCARDITIS PROPHYLAXIS

- Clinical indications
  - Prosthetic valve or prosthetic material in valve repair (MV ring)
  - Prior infective endocarditis
  - Completely repaired congenital heart disease if prosthetic material placed within last 6 months
  - Repaired congenital heart disease with residual defects
  - Unrepaired **cyanotic** congenital heart disease
    - VSD / ASD / PDA with L → R shunt does **not** require prophylaxis
  - Transplant with valvulopathy

- Procedures requiring consideration of prophylaxis
  - Dental procedures
  - Respiratory procedures requiring incision or biopsy
  - Bronchoscopy without biopsy does **not** require prophylaxis
  - GI / GU procedures → **no** indication for prophylaxis

- Antibiotic prophylaxis
  - All given as single doses 30–60 minutes prior to procedure
  - Preferred → amoxicillin 2 g PO
  - PCN allergic → clindamycin 600 mg PO or azithromycin 500 mg PO
  - Unable to take PO → ampicillin 2 g IV or cefazolin 1 g IV / IM
  - Unable to take PO and PCN allergic → cefazolin 1 g IV or clindamycin 600 mg IV / IM

DEVICE INFECTION

- Complete device removal is mandatory even for localized infections
- Typically treat with antibiotics for 7–14 days after device removed
- Reimplant on contralateral side after 72 hours of negative blood cultures
- LVAD Infection
  - *Staph aureus* is most common organism
  - Treat with parenteral antibiotics followed by oral suppression
  - Does not affect transplant outcomes

REFERENCES

1. Nishimura RA, Otto CM, Bonow RO, et al. 2017 AHA/ACC focused update of the 2014 AHA/ACC guideline for the management of patients with valvular heart disease: A report of the American College of Cardiology/American Heart Association Task Force on Clinical Practice Guidelines. *J Am Coll Cardiol.* 2017;70(2):252–289. (doi: 10.1016/j.jacc.2017.03.011)

2. Baddour LM, Wilson WR, Bayer AS, et al. Infective endocarditis in adults: diagnosis, antimicrobial therapy, and management of complications: A scientific statement for healthcare professionals from the American Heart Association. *Circulation.* 2015;132:1435–1486. (doi: 10.1161/CIR.0000000000000296)

3. Hyle EP, Hurtado RM, Gandhi RT. Chapter 29: Infective endocarditis, device infections, and cardiac manifestations of HIV. In: Gaggin HK, Januzzi JL. *MGH cardiology board review.* London: Springer-Verlag; 2013:486–504. (doi: 10.1007/978-1-4471-4483-0)

CHAPTER 12

HYPERTENSION

DEFINITIONS

Normal	< 120 / < 80
Elevated	120–129 / < 80
Stage 1	130–139 or 80–89
Stage 2	≥ 140 or ≥ 90

INTERVENTION

- Elevated / Stage 1 with ASCVD risk < 10%
  - 3–6 months of therapeutic lifestyle changes
  - Weight loss / exercise / sodium restriction (< 2400 mg/day) / potassium supplementation

- Stage 1 with ASCVD risk ≥ 10% and Stage 2
  - Start pharmacologic therapy and therapeutic lifestyle changes concurrently

- Stage 2 → Initiate therapy with two first-line agents from different classes

- First-line agents

- ACE/ARB, CCB, or thiazide
- **Always start ACE/ARB in patients with CKD**
- African American patients **without CKD,** CCB, or thiazide is preferred first-line therapy

TREATMENT GOAL

< 130/80

SECONDARY HYPERTENSION

- When to screen:
  - New onset HTN
  - Uncontrolled / drug-resistant (≥ 3 antihypertensives, including diuretic)
  - Age < 30
  - CAD / CKD / PAD
  - Albuminuria
  - Hypokalemia

- Conditions to initially screen for:
  - Renal artery stenosis
  - Primary aldosteronism
  - Obstructive sleep apnea
  - Drugs (NSAIDs / steroids / androgens / decongestants / caffeine / MAOI)

- Screen for other conditions only if suggested by specific clinical characteristics
  - Pheochromocytoma
  - Cushing disease
  - Adrenal hyperplasia
  - Hypothyroidism / hyperthyroidism
  - Aortic coarctation

SPECIFIC CAUSES OF SECONDARY HYPERTENSION

○ Renovascular
  - Progressive renal artery stenosis secondary to atherosclerosis → reduced intraglomerular pressure → activation of renin-angiotensin-aldosterone system
    - Medical therapy is treatment of choice for most
    - Reasonable to consider (IIb recommendation) renal artery angioplasty / stent placement for patients who fail medical therapy
      ○ Refractory HTN / worsening renal function / refractory heart failure

○ Primary aldosteronism
  - ↓ renin / ↑ aldosterone / hypokalemia
  - Diagnosis
    - Plasma aldosterone concentration (PAC) / plasma renin activity (PRA) ratio > 25 and plasma aldosterone concentration > 15 ng/dL
    - PRA typically less than 1.0 ng/dL
    - OK to continue ACE for initial PAC / PRA screening. Must d/c aldosterone antagonists
  - Confirmatory tests if PAC/PRA abnormal
    1. Urinary aldosterone > 12 mg/24 hours after 6 g/day sodium load
    2. Plasma Aldo > 10 ng/dL after 2L NS over 4 hours
    3. Captopril challenge
    - 25–50 mg captopril
      ○ Plasma aldo ↑ / plasma renin ↓

- If confirmatory test positive, perform abdominal CT to look for adrenal adenoma
- If CT suggests unilateral disease, perform adrenal vein sampling to confirm unilateral disease vs. bilateral (adrenal hyperplasia)
  - Surgical resection for unilateral disease
  - Aldosterone antagonists for bilateral disease
- OSA
  - Common cause of resistant HTN
  - Treat with CPAP / BiPAP
- Cushing disease
  - Excess cortisol → easy bruisability, proximal muscle weakness, hirsutism, HTN
  - Carney complex → hypercortisolism, myxoma, pigmented dermal lesions
  - Diagnosis
    - ↑ 24 hour urinary cortisol
    - Abnormal dexamethasone suppression test
  - Cause
    - ACTH producing pituitary adenoma (↑ ACTH / ↑ cortisol)
    - Adrenal adenoma (↓↓ ACTH / ↑ cortisol)
      - Both are treated surgically
- Coarctation of the aorta
  - See Chapter 17: Congenital Heart Disease – Simple Lesions

- Pheochromocytoma
  - Catecholamine-secreting tumor → episodic flushing, palpitations, severe HTN
  - Diagnosis
    - Screen with plasma metanephrines
    - Confirm with 24 hour urinary catecholamines and metanephrines
      - If positive → CT or MRI to localize the tumor
  - Treatment
    - Surgical resection
    - Need alpha- (phenoxybenzamine) and beta-blockade prior to surgery

RESISTANT HTN

- BP above goal despite 3 classes of antihypertensives (must include diuretic)
  - Consider addition of spironolactone

HYPERTENSIVE EMERGENCIES

- Hypertensive urgency
  - 180/120 – developing rapidly / no symptoms or end organ damage
    - Reinstitute or intensify oral therapy and arrange close outpatient follow-up
- Hypertensive emergency
  - > 180/120 with evidence of end organ damage
    - Retinal hemorrhage, acute renal failure, encephalopathy, angina, etc.
    - Reduce SBP no more than 25% in the first hour / 160/100 next 2–6 hours / lower BP to normal over next 24–48 hours
  - Avoid SBP < 160 acutely

- Aortic dissection
  - Lower SBP to < 120 mmHg within the first hour
    - Esmolol or labetalol is initial agent of choice
    - Nicardipine or nitroprusside if further blood pressure lowering required

HYPERTENSION IN PREGNANCY

- Gestational HTN
  - HTN developing after the 20th week of pregnancy / resolves within 12 weeks postpartum
  - Rx → labetalol, methyldopa, nifedipine
  - **ACE / ARB contraindicated** (risk of major congenital malformations)

- Preeclampsia
  - Gestational HTN + proteinuria (> 300 mg/24 hours)

REFERENCES

1. Whelton PK, Carey RM, Aronow WS, et al. 2017 ACC/AHA/AAPA/ABC/ACPM/AGS/APhA/ASH/ASPC/NMA/PCNA guideline for the prevention, detection, evaluation, and management of high blood pressure in adults. *J Am Coll Cardiol.* (2017). (doi: 10.1016/j.jacc.2017.11.006)

2. James PA, Oparil S, Carter BL, Cushman WC, et al. 2014 evidence-based guideline for the management of high blood pressure in adults: Report from the panel members appointed to the Eighth Joint National Committee (JNC 8). *JAMA.* 2014;311(5):507–520. (doi: 10.1001/jama.2013.284427)

3. Kendrick J, Chonchol M. Renal artery stenosis and chronic ischemic nephropathy: Epidemiology and diagnosis. *Adv Chronic Kidney Dis.* 2008;15:355–362. (doi: 10.1053/j.ackd.2008.07.004)

4. Mosso L, Carvajal C, Gonzalez A, et al. Primary aldosteronism and hypertensive disease. *Hypertension.* 2003;42:161–165. (doi: 10.1161/01.HYP.0000079505.25750.11)

5. Funder JW, Carey RM, Fardella C, et al. Case detection, diagnosis, and treatment of patients with primary aldosteronism: An endocrine society clinical practice guideline. *J Clin Endocrinol Metab.* 2008;93(9):3266–3281. (doi: 10.1210/jc.2008-0104)

6. Biller BM, Grossman AB, Stewart PM, et al. Treatment of adrenocorticotropin-dependent Cushing's syndrome: A consensus statement. *J Clin Endocrinol Metab.* 2008; 93:2454–2462. (doi: 10.1210/jc.2007-2734)

7. Orth DN. Cushing's syndrome. *N Engl J Med.* 1995;332:791–803. (doi: 10.1056/NEJM199506013322223)

8. Hogan MJ. Chapter 61: Hypertension. In: Murphy JG, Lloyd MA. *Mayo clinic cardiology concise textbook.* Rochester: Mayo Scientific Press; 2007:741–749.

9. Kostis WJ, Zusman RM. Chapter 5: Hypertension. In: Gaggin HK, Januzzi JL. *MGH cardiology board review.* London: Springer London; 2013:86–104. (doi: 10.1007/978-1-4471-4483-0)

10. Pacak K, Linehan WM, Eisenhofer G, et al. Recent advances in genetics, diagnosis, localization, and treatment of pheochromocytoma. *Ann Intern Med.* 2001;134:315-29. (doi: 10.7326/0003-4819-134-4-200102200-00016)

11. Calhoun DA, Jones D, Textor S, et al. Resistant hypertension: Diagnosis, evaluation, and treatment. A scientific statement from the American Heart Association Professional Education Committee of the Council for High Blood Pressure Research. *Circulation.* 2008;117:e510–e526. (doi: 10.1161/CIRCULATIONAHA.108.189141)

12. Mancia G, Fagard R, Narkiewicz K, et al. 2013 ESH/ESC Guidelines for the management of arterial hypertension: the Task Force for the management of arterial hypertension of the European Society of Hypertension (ESH) and of the European Society of Cardiology (ESC). *J Hypertens.* 2013;31:1281–1357. (doi: 10.1097/01.hjh.0000431740.32696.cc)

13. Johnson W, Nguyen ML, Patel R. Hypertension crisis in the emergency department. *Cardiol Clin.* 2012;30:533–543. (doi: 10.1016/j.ccl.2012.07.011)

14. Elliott WJ. Clinical features in the management of selected hypertensive emergencies. *Prog Cardiovasc Dis.* 2006;48:316–325. (doi: 10.1016/j.pcad.2006.02.004)

15. American College of Obstetricians and Gynecologists, Task Force on Hypertension in Pregnancy. Hypertension in pregnancy. Report of the American College of Obstetricians and Gynecologists' Task Force on Hypertension in Pregnancy. *Obstet Gynecol.* 2013;122:1122–1231. (doi: 10.1097/01.AOG.0000437382.03963.88)

SYNCOPE

PHYSIOLOGY OF VASOVAGAL SYNCOPE

○ ↓ venous return (venous pooling) → increased ventricular contractility → stimulates C-fibers (cardiac mechanoreceptors) → increased neural output to brainstem → fall in heart rate and peripheral vascular resistance

○ Vasovagal syncope is a diagnosis of exclusion and based primarily on the history
- Clear vasovagal syncope in a low-risk patient does not require further workup
- Carotid Doppler study is not useful in the workup of syncope because carotid disease is **not** associated with syncope

SUBCLAVIAN STEAL

○ Subclavian artery stenosis proximal to the origin of the ipsilateral vertebral artery
  - Increased circulatory demand in the ipsilateral arm (arm exercises) can → retrograde flow in the vertebral artery that shunts blood away from the cerebral circulation → neurologic symptoms
  - Diagnosed by CTA or color Doppler ultrasound

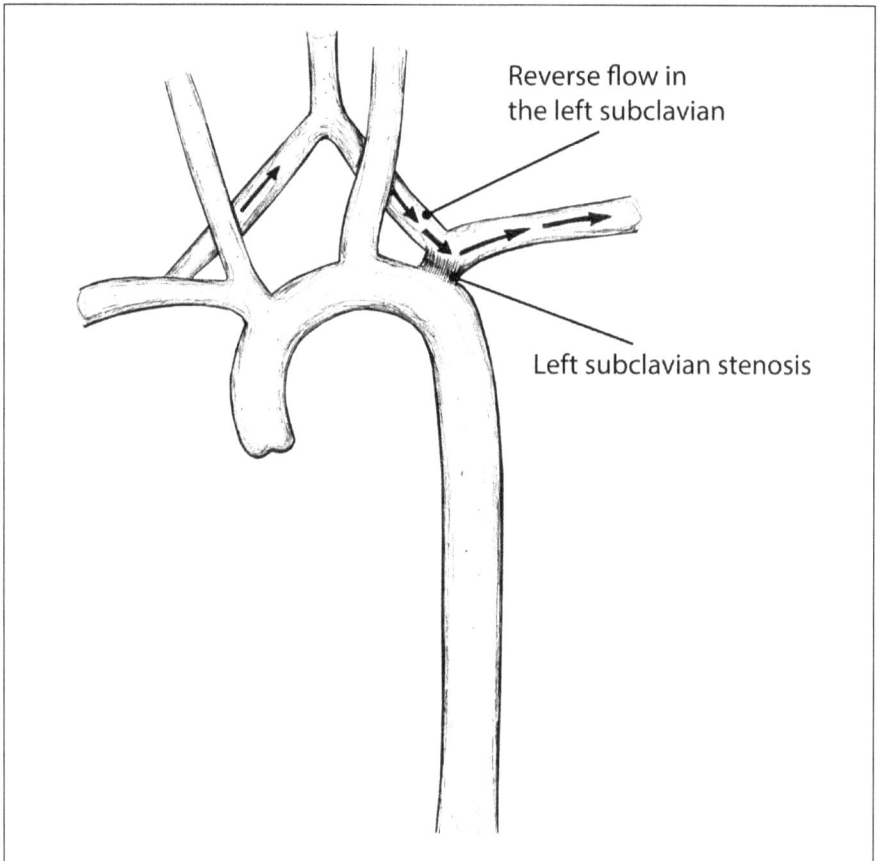

Figure 13.1 Mechanism of subclavian steal.

ORTHOSTATIC HYPOTENSION

○ Measure orthostatic vitals after **3 minutes** in each position:
  - Lying
  - Sitting
  - Standing

○ Positive if: SBP ↓ 20 mmHg / DBP ↓ 10 mmHg / HR ↑ 10–20 bpm

○ Treatment
  - Midodrine → vasoconstriction
  - Fludrocortisone ↓ volume expansion

CAROTID SINUS HYPERSENSITIVITY

○ Exaggerated response to carotid sinus baroreceptor stimulation → diminished cerebral circulation
  - Cardioinhibitory → Asystole ≥ 3 seconds
  - Vasodepressor → decrease in SBP ≥ 50 mmHg

○ Classic presentation is older male with symptoms while shaving, wearing a tight-collared shirt, etc.

○ PPM indications
  - Cardioinhibitory with symptomatic pause > 3 seconds or asymptomatic pause > 6 seconds → 2A indication
  - No role for pacing if strictly vasodepressor response

CLASS I INDICATIONS FOR TILT TABLE TESTING

○ Unexplained syncope in a high-risk setting (i.e., injury or occupational implication such as airline pilot)

○ Recurrent syncope in the absence of structural heart disease

EP STUDY IN THE EVALUATION OF SYNCOPE

○ Indications
  - Abnormal ECG suggesting disease of the conduction system
  - Supine syncope
  - Syncope with exertion
  - Known structural heart disease
  - Family history of sudden cardiac death
  - Syncope associated with palpitations or angina

○ Values to remember
  - Normal sinus node recovery time is < 3 seconds
  - Normal H-V interval is < 100 ms

○ Polymorphic VT / VF in a patient with underlying cardiomyopathy is **nondiagnostic**

REFERENCES

1. Moya A, Sutton R, Ammirati F, et al. Guidelines for the diagnosis and management of syncope (version 2009): The task force for the diagnosis and management of syncope of the European Society of Cardiology (ESC). *Eur Heart J.* 2009;30(21):2631–2671. (doi: 10.1093/eurheartj/ehp298)

2. Shen W-K, Sheldon RS, Benditt DG, et al. 2017 ACC/AHA/HRS guideline for the evaluation and management of patients with syncope: Executive summary: a report of the American College of Cardiology/American Heart Association Task Force on Clinical Practice Guidelines and the Heart Rhythm Society. *Circulation.* 2017;136:e25–e59. (doi: 10.1161/CIR.0000000000000498)

VASCULAR DISEASE

PERIPHERAL ARTERIAL DISEASE

$$ABI = \frac{\text{Ankle systolic BP}}{\text{Brachial systolic BP}}$$

- ○ Use highest brachial BP, either R or L
- ○ ABI typically reported for both R and L, but overall ABI is lowest value obtained
  - $\geq 1.40 \rightarrow$ non-compressible / uninterpretable
  - $1.0–1.39 \rightarrow$ normal
  - $0.41–0.99 \rightarrow$ mild to moderate PAD
  - $\leq 0.4 \rightarrow$ severe PAD
- ○ Medical management
  - Treat DM
    - Hb A1C goal < 7.0
  - CAD equivalent $\rightarrow$ statin (intensity based on age)
  - BP goal < 140/90
  - ASA or clopidogrel in all

- ○ Management of symptoms
  - ◉ Exercise is mainstay of treatment +/- cilostazol × 3–6 months
  - ◉ Interventional therapy only considered for life or work limiting symptoms after trial of exercise and medical therapy
    - • Essentially equivalent outcomes with endovascular vs. surgical approach
  - ◉ Acute limb ischemia
    - • Immediate parenteral anticoagulation followed by catheter-based thrombolysis

CAROTID ARTERIAL DISEASE

- ○ Guidelines do not specify a clear difference between stenting vs. endarterectomy
- ○ Asymptomatic disease
  - ◉ Consider revascularization if stenosis > 70% and low complication risk
- ○ Symptomatic disease (TIA / CVA within last 6 months)
  - ◉ Consider revascularization for angiographic lesion > 50% or > 70% by noninvasive imaging
- ○ Follow-up imaging
  - ◉ Asymptomatic disease
    - • Moderate (50%–69% stenosis) → reimage every 12 months
    - • Severe (70%–99% stenosis) → reimage at 6 months after initial diagnosis and then every 12 months
  - ◉ Following carotid intervention
    - • 6 months and 12 months after intervention, then every 12 months

ATHEROSCLEROTIC RENAL ARTERY STENOSIS

- Medical therapy is treatment of choice in all but very select population:
  - Bilateral renal artery stenosis with CHF
  - High-grade stenosis with resistant HTN despite 3+ drugs
- Fibromuscular dysplasia
  - Aggressive medical therapy is mainstay of treatment (ACE / ARB first-line)
  - **Angioplasty** only for resistant HTN (no role for stenting)

SUBCLAVIAN ARTERIAL DISEASE

- Subclavian stenosis proximal to the origin of the vertebral artery → vertebral steal during ipsilateral arm exercise (see Chapter 13: Syncope)
  - Due to metabolite induced vasodilation → reduced resistance in the subclavian artery distal to the stenosis → retrograde blood flow in the vertebral
    - May produce neurologic symptoms / presyncope
    - Patients with LIMA graft can experience angina if subclavian stenosis is proximal to the LIMA via retrograde flow in the LIMA by the same mechanism
  - Consider when > 15 mmHg BP difference between the arms
    - Confirm with Doppler ultrasound or angiography
  - Stenting is the preferred treatment
    - Indications: arm claudication, vertebral / coronary steal

DEEP VEIN THROMBOSIS

- Key to diagnosis is clinical likelihood
  - Clinical predictors
    - Active cancer
    - Immobilization
    - Recent major surgery
    - Swollen leg
    - Localized tenderness
    - Asymmetric calf swelling
    - Pitting edema
    - Collateral superficial veins
    - Hemoptysis
  - ANY above risk factor = intermediate or greater probability
    - Low probability
      - Presence of alternate diagnosis → no further testing
      - No alternate diagnosis → D-Dimer
        - Negative → no further testing
        - Positive → duplex
    - Intermediate / high probability → duplex

- Treatment
  - Provoked DVT → anticoagulate 3–6 months
  - Unprovoked DVT → anticoagulate 6 months – indefinite
  - 20–40 mmHg compression stockings for prevention of post-thrombotic syndrome

- Catheter associated thrombosis
  - Remove catheter / anticoagulate for 3 months

- Superficial venous thrombosis
  - Rx → NSAIDs / warm compresses

REFERENCES

1. Gerhard-Herman MD, Gornik HL, Barrett C, et al. 2016 AHA/ACC guideline on the management of patients with lower extremity peripheral artery disease: Executive summary: A report of the American College of Cardiology/American Heart Association Task Force on Clinical Practice Guidelines. *J Am Coll Cardiol.* 2017;69:1465–1508. (doi: 10.1016/j.jacc.2017.02.003)

2. Brott TG, Halperin JL, Abbara S, et al. 2011 ASA/ ACCF/AHA/ AANN/AANS/ ACR/CNS/SAIP/SCAI/SIR/ SNIS/SVM/SVS guideline on the management of patients with extracranial carotid and vertebral artery disease. *J Am Coll Cardiol.* 2011;57:1002–1044. (doi: 10.1016/j.jacc.2011.05.005)

3. Mohler III ER, Gornik HL, Gerhard-Herman M, et al. ACCF/ACR/ AIUM/ASE/ASN/ICAVL/SCAI/SCCT/SIR/SVM/SVS 2012 appro-priate use criteria for peripheral vascular ultrasound and physiological testing part I: Arterial ultrasound and physiological testing. *J Am Coll Cardiol.* 2012;60:242–276. (doi: 10.1016/j.jacc.2012.02.009)

4. Hirsch AT, Haskal ZJ, Hertzer NR, et al. ACC/AHA 2005 practice guidelines for the management of patients with peripheral arterial disease (lower extremity, renal, mesenteric, and abdominal aor-tic): A collaborative report from the American Association for Vascular Surgery/Society for Vascular Surgery, Society for Cardiovascular Angiography and Interventions, Society for Vascular Medicine and Biology, Society of Interventional Radiology, and the ACC/AHA Task Force on Practice Guidelines (Writing Committee to Develop Guidelines for the Management of Patients With Peripheral Arterial Disease). *Circulation.* 2006;113:e463–e654. (doi: 10.1161/CIRCULATIONAHA.106.174526)

5. Mazzolai L, Aboyans V, Ageno W, et al. Diagnosis and manage-ment of acute deep vein thrombosis: a joint consensus document from the european society of cardiology working groups of aorta and peripheral circulation and pulmonary circulation and right ventricular function. *Eur Heart J.* 2017;Feb 17:[Epub ahead of print]. (doi: 10.1093/eurheartj/ehx003)

CHAPTER 15

DISEASES OF THE AORTA

- ○ Normal aortic size
  - ⊛ Root < 4.0 cm
  - ⊛ Ascending aorta < 3.5 cm
  - ⊛ Descending aorta < 2.5 cm
  - ⊛ Abdominal aorta < 2.0 cm

- ○ Aneurysm → dilation involving all three layers of the vessel wall

- ○ Pseudoaneurysm → contained rupture

THORACIC AORTIC ANEURYSM (TAA)

- ○ Commonly associated with bicuspid aortic valve (BAV)
  - ⊛ All patients discovered to have BAV should have evaluation for TAA
    - • Transthoracic echo is initial screening test
      - ○ Dilated ascending aorta → CT or MRI to evaluate entire aorta

- ○ Commonly associated genetic syndromes
  - ◉ Marfan syndrome
    - Autosomal dominant / defect in fibrillin-1
    - Commonly associated with aortopathy / aortic valve disease / ocular, skeletal defects
  - ◉ Loeys-Dietz
    - **Bifid uvula**
  - ◉ Ehlers-Danlos
    - Autosomal dominant / defect in procollagen

- ○ Medical therapy
  - ◉ If aortic aneurysm detected by any imaging modality, full imaging study should be done
  - ◉ Yearly imaging after diagnosis
  - ◉ Echo or CT for all first degree relatives of anyone with TAA
  - ◉ Treat hypertension per guideline recommendations
    - Beta-blockers are first-line in patients with Marfan syndrome
  - ◉ Avoid heavy lifting or straining

- ○ Indications for repair
  - ◉ ≥ 5.5 cm (includes patients with BAV and no other risk factors)
  - ◉ ≥ 5.0 cm for Marfan / family history of aortic dissection
  - ◉ ≥ 4.5 cm undergoing cardiothoracic surgery for another indication
  - ◉ > 4.0 cm in Marfan patients considering pregnancy
  - ◉ ≥ 4.2–4.4 cm in Loeys-Dietz
  - ◉ Aortic arch ≥ 5.5 cm
  - ◉ Descending aorta ≥ 5.5–6.0 cm
    - Endovascular repair also an option for descending aorta

AORTIC DISSECTION

○ Intimal tear allowing penetration of blood into medial layer → second channel (false lumen)
  - Abrupt, sharp, tearing pain
    - Typically maximum pain at onset
  - BP difference > 20 mmHg considered significant
  - Classification of dissection
    - DeBakey I
      ○ Ascending + **arch** +/– descending
    - DeBakey II
      ○ Ascending **only**
    - Stanford A = DeBakey I or II
      ○ Ascending +/– arch
    - DeBakey III / Stanford B
      ○ Descending only

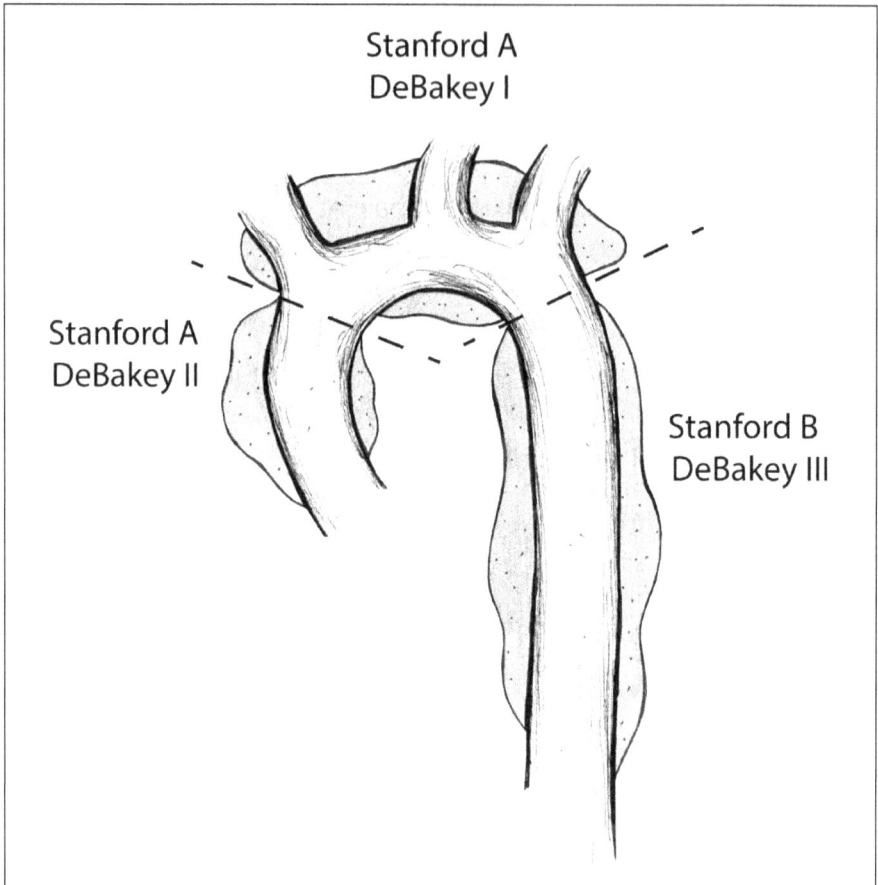

Figure 15.1 Stanford and Debakey classification schemes of aortic dissection.

○ Treatment
  - Type A / DeBakey I / II → surgical emergency
    • Preoperative coronary angiography typically **not** performed as it is an unnecessary delay to surgery
  - Type B / DeBakey III may be managed medically
    • Beta-blockers (labetalol) first-line to limit reflex tachycardia
    • Goal HR < 60 / SBP < 100–120 (acute and chronically)

- Intramural hematoma
  - Bleeding contained within the media of the aortic wall without communication with the aortic lumen
    - Due to vasa vasorum rupture or microscopic intimal tears
  - Treatment approach is identical to aortic dissection
- Penetrating atherosclerotic ulcer
  - Atherosclerotic plaque disrupts internal elastic lamina, allowing blood to penetrate aortic wall
  - Typically occurs in descending aorta
  - Typically managed medically
  - Large, expanding, or development of pseudoaneurysms may require intervention
    - Endovascular repair preferred
- Aortic transection
  - Most commonly occurs at ligamentum arteriosum due to deceleration injury
  - Surgical emergency

ABDOMINAL AORTIC ANEURYSM

- Males predominate (10:1)
- Major risk factors → atherosclerosis / smoking
- Screening
  - Males > 60 years old with first-degree relative with AAA
  - Males 65–74 years old with any history of smoking
- Medical treatment
  - Smoking cessation / statin / beta-blocker

- Monitoring
  - 3.0–3.4 cm → every 3 years
  - 3.5–4.4 cm → every 12 months
  - 4.5–5.4 cm → every 6 months

- Indications for repair
  - Male ≥ 5.5 cm / female ≥ 5.0 cm
  - Growth > 0.5 cm/year
  - Symptoms are always an indication for repair at any size

- Options for repair
  - Surgery → resect and replace with synthetic graft
  - Endovascular aortic aneurysm repair (EVAR)
    - Stent deployed proximal and distal to aneurysm site
      - → excludes aneurysm from aortic blood flow
    - Endoleak = persistent blood flow into aneurysm sac due to inability to completely exclude it from circulation
      - EVAR requires CT or MR imaging at 1 month, 6 months, and then yearly to exclude endoleak or graft migration
        - Inability to comply with follow-up requirements is an indication for open surgical repair

VASCULITIDES

- ○ Giant cell arteritis (temporal arteritis)
    - ● Associated with polymyalgia rheumatica
    - ● Develop thoracic aortic aneurysms as late complication
        - • Surveillance imaging for up to 10 years
    - ● Treat with high-dose steroids

- ○ Takayasu arteritis
    - ● Seen most commonly in East Asia / Africa
    - ● Females predominate
    - ● Granulomatous vasculitis affecting aorta / brachiocephalic / PA / coronary ostia
    - ● Initial nonspecific phase (fever, sweats, weight loss) then aneurysms or stenosis
    - ● Treated with high-dose steroids

REFERENCES

1. Hiratzka LF, Bakris GL, Beckman JA, et al. 2010 ACCF/AHA/AATS/ ACR/ASA/SCA/SCAI/SIR/STS/SVM guidelines for the diagnosis and management of patients with thoracic aortic disease: Executive summary: A report of the American College of Cardiology Foundation/American Heart Association Task Force on Practice Guidelines, American Association for Thoracic Surgery, American College of Radiology, American Stroke Association, Society of Cardiovascular Anesthesiologists, Society for Cardiovascular Angiography and Interventions, Society of Interventional Radiology, Society of Thoracic Surgeons, and Society for Vascular Medicine. *Circulation.* 2010;121:1544–1579. (doi: 10.1161/CIR.0b013e3181d47d48)

2. Hiratzka LF, Nishimura RA, Bonow RO, et al. Surgery for aortic dilatation in patients with bicuspid aortic valves: A statement of clarification from the American College of Cardiology/American Heart Association Task Force on Clinical Practice Guidelines. *J Am Coll Cardiol.* 2016;67:724–731. (doi: 10.1016/j.jacc.2015.11.006)

3. Gerhard-Herman MD, Gornik HL, Barrett C, et al. 2016 AHA/ACC guideline on the management of patients with lower extremity peripheral artery disease: A report of the American College of Cardiology/American Heart Association Task Force on Clinical Practice Guidelines. *J Am Coll Cardiol.* 2017;69:e71–126. (doi: 10.1016/j.jacc.2016.11.007)

4. Rooke TW, Hirsch AT, Misra S, et. al. ACCF/AHA focused update of the guideline for the management of patients with peripheral artery disease (updating the 2005 guideline): A report of the American College of Cardiology Foundation/American Heart Association Task Force on Practice Guidelines. *Circulation.* 2011;124:2020–2045. (doi: 10.1161/CIR.0b013e31822e80c3)

5. Wennberg PW. Chapter 53: Vasculitis. In: Murphy JG, Lloyd MA. *Mayo clinic cardiology concise textbook.* 3rd ed. Rochester: Mayo Clinic Scientific Press; 2007:663–672.

CHAPTER 16

HEART DISEASE IN WOMEN AND PREGNANCY

PRIMARY PREVENTION

- ○ Hormone replacement therapy carries a Class III indication

- ○ Antioxidants / vitamin E and C / beta carotene / folic acid all carry Class III indication

- ○ No indication for routine ASA without risk factors

- ○ Statins have Class I indication post-MI even with normal lipids

PHYSIOLOGY OF PREGNANCY

- ○ Increased blood volume → increased preload

- ○ Decreased systemic vascular resistance → decreased afterload

- ○ Increased heart rate

○ Increased stroke volume
  ◦ Peaks around 31 weeks then falls due to decreased venous return related to caval compression

CONDITIONS WITH INCREASED MATERNAL RISK DURING PREGNANCY

○ History of CHF / CVA / TIA / symptomatic arrhythmia

○ Aortic stenosis < 1.5 cm² / Mitral stenosis < 2.0 cm² / LVOT gradient > 30 mmHg

○ Ejection fraction < 40%

○ History of peripartum cardiomyopathy → high risk of recurrence
  ◦ Future pregnancies should be avoided / terminated

VALVULAR HEART DISEASE IN PREGNANCY

○ Mitral regurgitation
  ◦ Typically well tolerated during pregnancy
  ◦ ↓ SVR typically offsets ↑ blood volume

- ○ Mitral stenosis
  - ● ↑ blood volume / tachycardia during pregnancy can worsen symptoms
  - ● Mild – moderate mitral stenosis typically well tolerated
  - ● Severe mitral stenosis requires close monitoring
    - Afib is common
      - ○ Digoxin, beta-blockers, diuretics OK for medical management
      - ○ Cardioversion for hemodynamic instability
    - Percutaneous valvuloplasty during pregnancy may be required for persistent symptoms / pulmonary artery systolic pressure > 50 mmHg
  - ● Antibiotics for endocarditis prophylaxis recommended at delivery
- ○ Aortic insufficiency
  - ● Typically well tolerated
  - ● ↓ systemic vascular resistance / tachycardia of pregnancy typically → decreased regurgitant volume
  - ● Endocarditis prophylaxis recommended at delivery
- ○ Aortic stenosis
  - ● Typically due to bicuspid aortic valve
  - ● Usually well-tolerated
    - Increased blood volume can worsen effects of stenosis
  - ● Severe stenosis (mean gradient > 50 mmHg, valve area < 1.0 cm^2) with symptoms requires balloon valvuloplasty prior to delivery
  - ● Antibiotics for endocarditis prophylaxis recommended at delivery

CONGENITAL HEART DISEASE IN PREGNANCY

- Atrial septal defect
  - Low maternal risk
  - Small risk of paradoxical embolism
  - Does not require antibiotics at delivery

- Ventricular septal defect
  - Low maternal risk (unless associated pulmonary HTN / Eisenmenger syndrome → high risk)
  - Antibiotics for endocarditis prophylaxis recommended at delivery

- Patent ductus arteriosus
  - Low maternal risk
  - Does not require endocarditis prophylaxis

- Coarctation of the aorta
  - Moderate maternal risk
    - Increased risk of HTN / CHF / intrauterine growth retardation
  - Association with bicuspid aortic valve and intracerebral aneurysms
    - Coarctation alone does not require antibiotic prophylaxis but bicuspid aortic valve should receive antibiotics

- Marfan syndrome
    - High maternal risk → 1% risk of fatal complications
  - Aortic root > 4.0 cm should be repaired prior to pregnancy
    - 10% risk of rupture for root > 4.5 cm

- Root monitored throughout pregnancy by echocardiography
  - Dilation during pregnancy may require termination
- Beta-blockers decrease risk of aortic rupture
- Delivery via C-section with general anesthesia to keep BP low
- Antibiotic prophylaxis at delivery recommended

○ Eisenmenger's syndrome
- Very high maternal risk → 30%–50% maternal mortality risk
- Typically due to uncorrected ASD / VSD / PDA → increased pulmonary pressures that eventually exceed systemic pressures → shunt reversal, becoming right to left → cyanosis
- Pregnancy should be avoided / terminated
- High thromboembolic risk
  - Anticoagulate third trimester through 1 month postpartum
- C-section should be avoided
  - General anesthesia lowers systemic vascular resistance, worsens right → left shunt

○ Tetralogy of Fallot
- Low maternal risk if repaired with no residual lesions
- Pregnancy should be terminated if unrepaired

○ Ebstein's anomaly
- High risk of SVT (WPW)

HYPERTENSION IN PREGNANCY

○ Chronic hypertension
  - BP > 140/90 prior to pregnancy or by 20th week

○ Gestational hypertension
  - HTN (BP > 140/90) developing after 20th week / resolves by 12 weeks postpartum

○ Treatment
  - Treat when diastolic pressure > 110 mmHg
  - Primary agents
    • Methyldopa
    • Labetalol
    • Nicardipine
  - Second line agents
    • Amlodipine
    • Beta-blockers
      ○ Avoid while breast feeding → fetal bradycardia
    • Hydralazine
    • HCTZ
  - ACE / ARB **contraindicated** in all circumstances due to teratogenic potential

○ Preeclampsia
  - HTN with proteinuria (> 300 mg/24 hours)
  - Start antihypertensive treatment when SBP > 160 mmHg or DBP > 105 mmHg
  - Require immediate delivery for seizures, cerebral hemorrhage, pulmonary edema, liver / renal failure, HELLP syndrome (Hemolysis, Elevated LFTs, Low Platelets)

ANTIARRHYTHMICS

Adenosine safe in pregnancy / all others used with caution

ANTICOAGULATION IN PREGNANCY

- ○ Weeks 1–12 → unfractionated heparin (UFH) or low molecular weight heparin (LMWH)
  - Does not cross placenta / less teratogenicity
- ○ Weeks 12–35 → warfarin
- ○ Week 35 – delivery → UFH / or plan for C-section week 38 with brief interruption of warfarin
- ○ If warfarin dose ≤ 5 mg daily it is **probably safe** in weeks 1–12 as well
- ○ If preferred, UFH or LMWH can be used throughout pregnancy

REFERENCES

1. Canobbio MM, Warnes CA, Aboulhosn J, et al; on behalf of the American Heart Association Council on Cardiovascular and Stroke Nursing; Council on Clinical Cardiology; Council on Cardiovascular Disease in the Young; Council on Functional Genomics and Translational Biology; and Council on Quality of Care and Outcomes Research. Management of pregnancy in patients with complex congenital heart disease: A scientific statement for healthcare professionals from the American Heart Association. *Circulation.* 2017;135:e1–e38. (doi: 10.1161/CIR.0000000000000458)

2. Regitz-Zagrosek V, Lundqvist CB, Claudio Borghi C, et al. ESC Guidelines on the management of cardiovascular diseases during pregnancy. *Eur Heart J.* 2011;32:3147–3197. (doi: 10.1093/eurheartj/ehr218)

3. Greutmann M, Pieper PG. Pregnancy in women with congenital heart disease. *Eur Heart J. 2015*;36:2491–2499. (doi: 10.1093/eurheartj/ehv288)

4. Brickner ME, Cardiovascular management in pregnancy. *Circulation.* 2014;130:273–282. (doi: 10.1161/CIRCULATIONAHA.113.002105)

5. Gilstrap GL, Wood MJ. Chapter 12: Cardiovascular disease in women and pregnancy. In: Gaggin HK, Januzzi JL. *MGH cardiology board review.* London: Springer London; 2013:205–223. (doi: 10.1007/978-1-4471-4483-0)

ADULT CONGENITAL HEART DISEASE – SIMPLE LESIONS

LEFT-TO-RIGHT SHUNT LESIONS

○ Atrial septal defect (ASD)

1. Secundum
   - Most common (65%)
   - ECG → RBBB with **right** axis deviation
   - Wide, fixed split S2

2. Primum
   - ECG → RBBB with **left** axis deviation
   - Wide, fixed split S2
   - Commonly associated with cleft mitral valve

3. Sinus venosus
   - Associated with anomalous pulmonary venous drainage

4. Coronary sinus
   - Rare
   - Associated with other complex congenital lesions

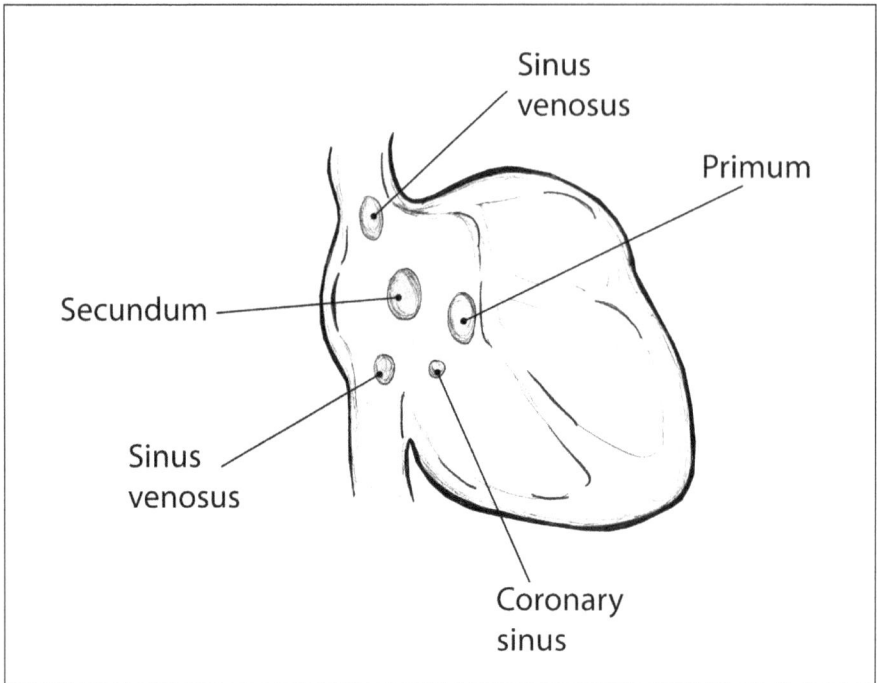

Figure 17.1 Simple atrial septal defects.

○ All ASDs result in increased RA/RV blood flow
  ● Untreated, can ultimately lead to Eisenmenger's syndrome

○ Indication for closure
  ● RA / RV enlargement with or without symptoms
  ● Uncomplicated secundum ASDs may be closed percutaneously
    • All others closed surgically

○ Ventricular septal defect (VSD)
1. Membranous / perimembranous
   ● Most common (60%–70%)
2. Muscular
3. Supracristal / outlet
   ● Frequently see associated aortic insufficiency
4. AV canal / inlet
   ● Associated with cleft mitral valve / primum ASD / Down syndrome

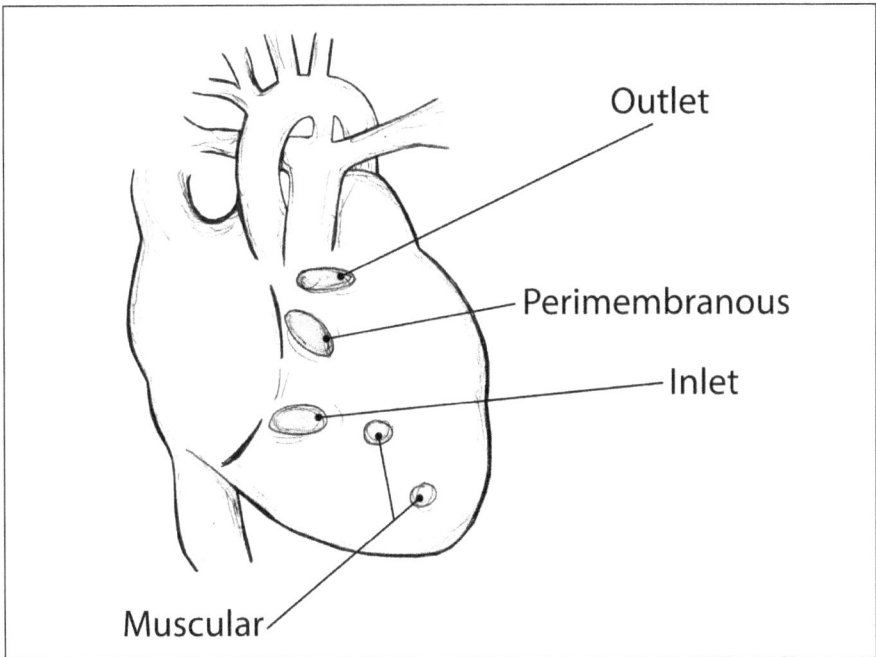

Figure 17.2 Simple ventricular septal defects.

○ VSDs → increased volume to LA / LV
   ● Small, restrictive VSDs rarely require treatment and frequently close spontaneously
○ Indications for closure
   ● Qp : Qs ≥ 2.0
   ● History of endocarditis
   ● LV enlargement

- Patent ductus arteriosus (PDA)
  - Ductus arteriosus connects distal aorta (typically just distal to left subclavian) to left pulmonary artery in utero
    - Diverts blood from the nonfunctioning pulmonary circuit to the aorta
    - Typically closes shortly after birth
  - Pulmonary vascular resistance drops at birth → left-to-right shunt
    - Increased pulmonary blood flow bypasses the RV and → LA / LV volume overload
  - Continuous "machinery" murmur
  - Eisenmenger's physiology can reverse the shunt to right → left
    - Presents with cyanosis of the feet / normal right hand / +/– left hand
- Management
  - Percutaneous or surgical closure for any of the following:
    - LA / LV enlargement
    - Pulmonary hypertension with **L → R** shunt
      - If Eisenmenger's physiology develops, care is strictly palliative
    - Endarteritis

OBSTRUCTIVE LESIONS

○ Bicuspid aortic valve
  ● Associated with coarctation of the aorta and cerebral aneurysms

○ Subaortic membrane
  ● Balloon dilation rarely successful
  ● Surgical indications
    • Peak gradient > 50 mmHg
    • Mean gradient > 30 mmHg
    • Left ventricular end systolic dimension ≥ 50 mm
    • Ejection fraction < 55%

○ Coarctation of the aorta
  ● Narrowing at the site of the ligamentum arteriosum (remnant of the ductus arteriosus) near the origin of the left subclavian
  ● Very commonly seen in association with bicuspid aortic valve (50%–60%)
  ● Frequent association with circle of Willis aneurysms
    • All patients diagnosed with coarctation should have screening CT or MRI to exclude cerebral aneurysm
  ● Collateral circulation via the intercostal arteries may reduce gradient across the coarct site
  ● Radial – femoral pulse delay is classic exam finding
    • BP difference > 20 mmHg between arms and legs consistent with coarct
  ● Indication for repair (surgical or percutaneous)
    • Peak to peak catheterization gradient ≥ 20 mmHg
  ● Reevaluate by CT or MRI a minimum of every 5 years following repair to exclude aneurysm formation or new obstruction

- ○ Pulmonic stenosis
  - ◉ Systolic ejection sound
    - Closer to S1 = more severe
    - **Only** right heart sound that **decreases** with inspiration
    - A2–P2 delay ↑ with ↑ severity
      - ○ Increased pulmonic ejection time
  - ◉ Treatment
    - Balloon valvotomy is treatment of choice
    - Indications
      - ○ Asymptomatic with peak doppler gradient > 60 mmHg or mean > 40 mmHg
      - ○ Symptomatic with peak gradient > 50 mmHg or mean > 30 mmHg

REFERENCES

1. Warnes CA, Williams RG, Bashore TM, et al. ACC/AHA 2008 guidelines for the management of adults with congenital heart disease: A report of the American College of Cardiology/American Heart Association Task Force on Practice Guidelines (Writing Committee to Develop Guidelines for the Management of Adults With Congenital Heart Disease). *Circulation.* 2008;118:2395–2451. (doi: 10.1161/CIRCULATIONAHA.108.190811)

2. Yeh DD, Liberthson RR, Bhatt AB et al. Chapter 21: Adult congenital heart disease (ACHD). In: Gaggin HK, Januzzi JL. *MGH cardiology board review.* London: Springer London; 2013:345–77. (doi: 10.1007/978-1-4471-4483-0)

3. Krasuski RA, Majdalany DS. Chapter 23: Congenital heart disease in the adult. In: Griffin BP, Kapadia SR, Rimmerman CM. *The Cleveland clinic cardiology board review.* 2nd ed. Philadelphia: Lippincott Williams & Wilkins; 2013:264–276.

4. Bhatt AB, Foster E, Kuehl K, et al. on behalf of the American Heart Association Council on Clinical Cardiology. Congenital heart disease in the older adult: A scientific statement from the American Heart Association. *Circulation.* 2015;131:1884–1931. (doi: 10.1161/CIR.0000000000000204)

CHAPTER 18

ADULT CONGENITAL HEART DISEASE – COMPLEX LESIONS

CONGENITAL CORONARY ANOMALIES

○ Anomalous left coronary artery from pulmonary artery
   - Few survive to adulthood without intervention
      • Rarely, coronary collateral flow allows survival undetected to adulthood
   - Treatment is coronary reimplantation

○ Anomalous coronaries coursing between aorta and pulmonary artery
   - Either left or right coronary can arise from contralateral sinus of Valsalva and travel anterior to the aorta and posterior to the pulmonary artery
      • Vessel is at risk for compression between aorta and pulmonary artery
   - Class I indications for surgical revascularization:
      • Left main traveling between aorta and pulmonary artery
      • Right coronary only if evidence of ischemia

CORONARY AV FISTULA

- ○ Most can be followed clinically
- ○ Coiling considered for large fistulas resulting in ischemia

EISENMENGER SYNDROME

- ○ Uncorrected L → R shunt leads to progressive ↑ in pulmonary vascular resistance
  - Eventually leads to shunt reversal (becomes R → L)
  - No effective medical therapy once shunt reversal occurs
    - Only definitive treatment is heart-lung transplant
  - Pregnancy **strictly contraindicated**
  - Need endocarditis prophylaxis

TETRALOGY OF FALLOT (TOF)

1. Right ventricular outflow obstruction

2. Ventricular septal defect

3. Overriding aorta

4. Right ventricular hypertrophy

- ○ Commonly associated with right-sided aortic arch
  - Cyanosis and right-sided aortic arch → consider TOF

- ○ ECG → RBBB with RVH
- ○ Palliative repairs
  - Provide pulmonary blood flow in the setting of RVOT obstruction but do not address any of the lesions themselves
    - Blalock-Taussig shunt
      - ○ R or L subclavian to branch PA
    - Rastelli procedure
      - ○ Valved conduit from RV to main PA
- ○ Complete repair is now usually performed in early childhood
- ○ Post-repair complications
  - Pulmonic insufficiency is most common
    - Valve replacement indicated in the setting of severe PI and any of the following:
      - ○ Symptoms / reduced functional capacity (only Class I indication)
      - ○ RV dysfunction / dilation (IIa)
      - ○ Atrial or ventricular arrhythmias (IIa)
      - ○ Moderate to severe TR (IIa)

TRANSPOSITION OF THE GREAT ARTERIES (TGA)

- D-transposition
  - Great vessels arise from the incorrect ventricle
    - Systemic venous return → RA → RV → aorta
    - Pulmonary venous return → LA → LV → PA
    - Aorta from RV / PA from LV → parallel circulation
    - Must be some mixing of oxygenated blood for survival (ASD, VSD, PDA)
      - Rashkind balloon atrial septostomy
        - ‣ Allows mixing of oxygenated blood until definitive repair can be performed
  - Arterial switch (Jatene procedure) is the definitive repair most commonly performed today
    - Aorta from LV / PA from RV
    - Normal exam / ECG
  - Senning / Mustard procedure performed until 1980s
    - Atrial switch
      - Systemic venous return baffled to LA
        - ‣ LA → LV → PA
      - Pulmonary venous return baffled to RA
        - ‣ RA → RV → aorta
    - RV becomes the systemic ventricle and will ultimately fail
      - Transplant is only treatment option when RV fails

- L-transposition (congenitally corrected TGA)
  - Atria and great arteries are "switched" →
    "corrected" blood flow
  - Systemic venous return → RA → MV → LV → PA
  - Pulmonary venous return → LA → TV → RV →
    aorta
    - Blood is oxygenated and distributed normally
      but the RV is the systemic ventricle
  - Consider L-transposition in any young patient
    with unexplained **complete heart block**
  - Transplant is ultimate treatment for RV failure
    unresponsive to medical therapy

EBSTEIN'S ANOMALY

- Characterized by apical displacement of the
  tricuspid valve
  - Echocardiography is diagnostic modality of choice

- Commonly associated with PFO / ASD
  - Risk of paradoxical embolism

- WPW present in approximately 25% with Ebstein's
  anomaly
  - Multiple bypass tracts are common and make
    arrhythmia management difficult

- Surgical intervention is highly individualized

TRICUSPID ATRESIA / SINGLE VENTRICLE

○ Surgical therapies
- PA banding
  - Protects the pulmonary circuit in patients with no limitation on pulmonary flow and large left → right shunts
- Glenn procedure (hemi-Fontan)
  - Directly connects SVC to R PA
    - ○ Bypasses right heart
- Fontan procedure
  - Systemic venous flow routed to the PA without passing through RV
    - ○ Anastomosed either directly to PA or via RA

DEXTROCARDIA

○ ECG → inverted P/QRS/T in I, aVL with reverse R-wave progression

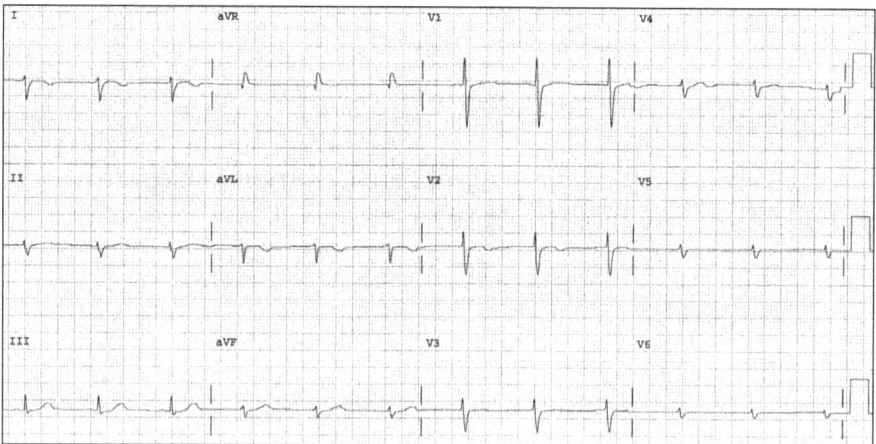

Figure 18.1 Dextrocardia.
Used with permission from Podrid P, Malhotra R, Kakar R, Noseworthy PA. *Podrid's Real-World ECGs: A Master's Approach to the Art and Practice of Clinical ECG Interpretation, Volume 6.* Minneapolis, MN: Cardiotext Publishing; 2016.

○ Distinguish from limb lead reversal
  ◉ Inverted P/QRS/T with **normal** R-wave progression

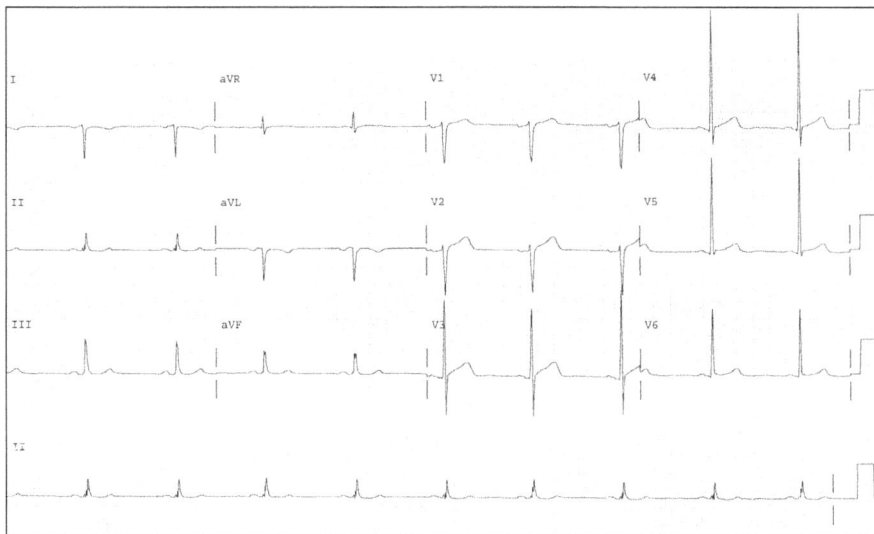

Figure 18.2 Limb lead reversal.
Used with permission from Podrid P, Malhotra R, Kakar R, Noseworthy PA. *Podrid's Real-World ECGs: A Master's Approach to the Art and Practice of Clinical ECG Interpretation, Volume 1.* Minneapolis, MN: Cardiotext Publishing; 2013.

CONGENITAL SURGERIES TO KNOW

○ Blalock-Taussig shunt
  ◉ Subclavian artery to branch PA

○ Waterston shunt
  ◉ Ascending aorta to PA

○ Potts shunt
  ◉ Descending aorta to PA

○ Mustard / Senning
  ◉ Atrial switch for D-transposition
  ◉ Systemic venous return baffled to LA → LV → PA
  ◉ Pulmonary venous return baffled to RA → RV → aorta

- Jatene
  - Arterial switch for D-transposition
  - Definitive treatment for D-transposition
    - Aorta reattached to LVOT / PA reattached to RVOT
- Glenn shunt
  - SVC to R PA
- Fontan procedure
  - SVC or RA anastomosed directly to PA
- Rastelli procedure
  - RV to PA conduit
  - Bypasses hypoplastic proximal PA
- PA banding
  - Reduces PA blood flow until definitive repair can be performed
  - Used when large L → R shunt overloads pulmonary circuit

CONGENITAL SYNDROMES AND ASSOCIATIONS TO KNOW

- Holt-Oram syndrome
  - ASD associated with abnormalities of the hand / radius
- Williams syndrome
  - Supravalvular aortic stenosis
  - Short / mental retardation
- Noonan syndrome
  - Short / pectus excavatum / mental retardation / hypertrophic cardiomyopathy / pulmonic stenosis

- ○ Down syndrome
  - ● ASD / VSD / TOF / PDA
- ○ Turner syndrome
  - ● Females / amenorrhea / bicuspid aortic valve / coarctation of the aorta
- ○ Congenital rubella
  - ● Deafness / ocular defects / PDA
- ○ Kartagener's syndrome
  - ● Sinusitis / bronchiectasis / dextrocardia
- ○ LEOPARD syndrome
  - ● L – Lentigines
  - ● E – ECG (conduction abnormalities)
  - ● O – Ocular
  - ● P – Pulmonic stenosis
  - ● A – Abnormal genitals
  - ● R – Retardation of growth
  - ● D – Deafness

REFERENCES

1. Warnes CA, Williams RG, Bashore TM, et al. ACC/AHA 2008 guidelines for the management of adults with congenital heart disease: A report of the American College of Cardiology/American Heart Association Task Force on Practice Guidelines (Writing Committee to Develop Guidelines for the Management of Adults With Congenital Heart Disease). *Circulation.* 2008;118:2395–2451. (doi: 10.1161/CIRCULATIONAHA.108.190811)

2. Yeh DD, Liberthson RR, Bhatt AB et al. Chapter 21: Adult congenital heart disease (ACHD). In: Gaggin HK, Januzzi JL. *MGH cardiology board review.* London: Springer London; 2013:345–77. (doi: 10.1007/978-1-4471-4483-0)

3. Krasuski RA, Majdalany DS. Chapter 23: Congenital heart disease in the adult. In: Griffin BP, Kapadia SR, Rimmerman CM. *The Cleveland clinic cardiology board review.* 2nd ed. Philadelphia: Lippincott Williams & Wilkins; 2013:264–276.

4. Bhatt AB, Foster E, Kuehl K, et al. on behalf of the American Heart Association Council on Clinical Cardiology. Congenital heart disease in the older adult: A scientific statement from the American Heart Association. *Circulation.* 2015;131:1884–1931. (doi: 10.1161/CIR.0000000000000204)

PULMONARY HYPERTENSION

○ Pulmonary hypertension
  ◦ Mean pulmonary artery pressure (mPAP)
    > 25 mmHg (by cath)

○ Pulmonary arterial hypertension
  ◦ Elevated pulmonary resistance due to restricted
    blood flow through the pulmonary circulation
    • Mean PAP > 25 mmHg / Pulmonary capillary
      wedge pressure (PCWP) or left ventricular
      end diastolic pressure (LVEDP) ≤ 15 mmHg /
      pulmonary vascular resistance (PVR)
      > 3 Wood units (WU)
    • PCWP or LVEDP > 15 mmHg / PVR < 3 is
      consistent with post-capillary (passive)
      pulmonary HTN
    • PVR = mPAP – mPCWP / cardiac output

WHO CLASSIFICATION

I – Pulmonary arterial HTN
  - Collagen vascular disease / HIV / drugs / thyroid disease / cirrhosis / pulmonary veno-occlusive

II – Pulmonary HTN related to left heart / valvular disease

III – Pulmonary HTN associated with lung disease and / or hypoxia
  - COPD / obstructive sleep apnea / interstitial lung disease / altitude

IV – Chronic thrombotic / embolic disease
  - Pulmonary emboli

V – Miscellaneous
  - Sarcoid
  - Any remaining condition not qualifying for one of the preceding four categories

WORKUP OF PULMONARY HYPERTENSION

Consider all of the following in anyone with newly diagnosed pulmonary hypertension:
  - ANA / RF / LFTs / HIV
  - Sleep study
  - PFTs
  - V/Q scan

RIGHT HEART CATHETERIZATION

○ Only indicated for group I patients
○ Vasodilator testing
  - Nitric oxide / adenosine / epoprostenol can all be used
  - Criteria defining response to vasodilator challenge
    - Decreased mPAP ≥ 10 mmHg **and** PA systolic ≤ 40 mmHg **without** fall in cardiac output (CO), **or:**
    - > 20% reduction in mPAP and PVR without fall in CO
  - PCWP > 15 mmHg and:
    - PVR < 3 WU → passive pulmonary HTN
      - o Diurese / treat left heart condition (typically CHF)
        - ‣ PVR > 3 WU
      - o No change in PVR with ↓ PCWP → fixed pulmonary HTN
      - o ↓ PVR with ↓ PCWP → Reactive pulmonary HTN
        - ‣ Appropriate for vasodilator therapy

GROUP I TREATMENT

○ Avoid pregnancy / high altitude

○ Oxygen therapy for saturation < 92%

○ These patients are typically anticoagulated due to high thromboembolic risk
- Warfarin is drug of choice / role of the novel oral anticoagulants is unknown

○ High-risk criteria:
- 6-minute walk < 165 m / SvO_2 < 60% / RV dysfunction / RA pressure > 14 mmHg / elevated BNP / elevated troponin

○ Responders to vasoreactivity testing treated with calcium channel blockers as first-line therapy
- Avoid verapamil due to negative inotropic effects

○ Non-high risk non-responders treated with PDE-5 or endothelin receptor antagonist
- 8PDE-5
  - Sildenafil
  - Tadalafil
- Endothelin receptor antagonists
  - Bosentan → check LFTs every 3 months
  - Ambrisentan
- High risk → prostacyclins
  - Epoprostenol
  - Treprostinil
  - Iloprost

- ○ Surgical interventions
  - ◉ Atrial septostomy
    - Only indicated as bridge to transplant in severe pulmonary HTN with intractable right heart failure despite maximum medical therapy
  - ◉ Transplant only indicated in the setting of intractable RV failure with **no other** end organ damage

GROUP II TREATMENT

- ○ Optimizing heart failure treatment is the mainstay of therapy
- ○ No role for PDE-5, endothelin antagonists, or prostacyclin

GROUP III TREATMENT

- ○ Treat hypoxia
- ○ If pulmonary HTN is severe, COPD, ILD, or sleep apnea is **rarely** the sole cause → always need to investigate for other causes

GROUP IV TREATMENT

- ○ V/Q scan better than CT to diagnose **chronic** thromboembolic disease
- ○ Pulmonary angiography remains the gold standard
- ○ Treatment
  - ◉ Diuretics / oxygen / lifelong anticoagulation
  - ◉ Thromboendarterectomy is the definitive treatment

REFERENCES

1. Galie N, Humbert M, Vachiery JL, et al. 2015 ESC/ERS guidelines for the diagnosis and treatment of pulmonary hypertension. The Joint Task Force for the Diagnosis and Treatment of Pulmonary Hypertension of the European Society of Cardiology (ESC) and the European Respiratory Society (ERS). *Eur Heart J.* 2016;37:67–119. (doi: 10.1093/eurheartj/ehv317)

2. McLaughlin VV, Archer SL, Badesch DB, et al. ACCF/AHA 2009 expert consensus document on pulmonary hypertension: A report of the American College of Cardiology Foundation Task Force on Expert Consensus Documents and the American Heart Association. *Circulation.* 2009;119:2250–2294. (doi: 10.1161/CIRCULATIONAHA.109.192230)

3. Clarke J, Lewis GD. Chapter 22: Pulmonary hypertension. In: Gaggin HK, Januzzi JL. *MGH cardiology board review.* London: Springer London; 2013:378–393. (doi: 10.1007/978-1-4471-4483-0)

CHAPTER 20

RESTRICTION / CONSTRICTION / TAMPONADE

RESTRICTIVE AND INFILTRATIVE CARDIOMYOPATHY

○ Normal or decreased ventricular volume with significant bi-atrial enlargement

○ Restrictive filling
- Deceleration time < 160 ms
- E/A ≥ 2
- e′ < 10 cm/s
- LA volume index > 34 mL/m²
- Invasive hemodynamics → Dip and plateau / square root sign (also seen in constrictive pericarditis)
  - Rapid early decline in ventricular pressure at onset of diastole with rapid rise to plateau in mid-diastole
    - Manifests as rapid y descent on RA tracing

- ○ Amyloidosis
  - Significant LVH with normal ECG voltage
  - Echo → severely dilated atria with LVH / normal to small LV cavity size
  - Treatment → transplant

CONSTRICTIVE PERICARDITIS

- ○ Calcified pericardium prevents transmission of intrathoracic pressures to the heart
  - Inspiration → decreased intrathoracic pressure → decreased pulmonary venous pressure but no change in LA pressure → decreased PV – LA driving pressure
    - Allows for preferential right heart filling → interventricular septum shifts to the left (because RV constrained by fibrotic pericardium)
      - ○ Leads to discordant RV / LV fillings (ventricular interdependence)
- ○ Invasive hemodynamics
  - Rapid early diastolic filling → steep y descent, limited later in diastole by stiff, fibrotic pericardium → Dip and plateau / square root sign
- ○ Management
  - Do not diagnose in the immediate post-op setting → likely to recover within weeks to months of surgery
  - Initial treatment is relief of congestion → diuretics
  - Consider pericardial stripping for refractory symptoms / low output

DISTINGUISHING CONSTRICTION FROM RESTRICTION

Restriction	Constriction
Reduced e' (< 10 cm/s)	NL / ↑ e'
RVSP > 55 mmHg	RVSP < 55 mmHg
LVEDP – RVEDP > 5 mmHg	LVEDP-RVEDᵒP < 5 mmHg
Concordant RV / LV pressures with respiration	**Discordant** RV / LV pressures with respiration

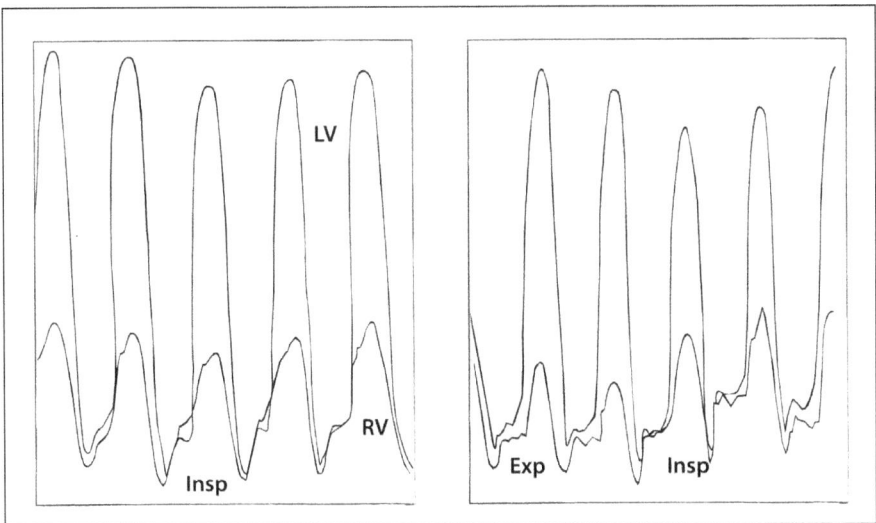

Figure 20.1 Invasive hemodynamics of restriction vs. constriction. *Note:* Concordant RV / LV pressures with respiration in restrictive cardiomyopathy vs. discordant pressures in constrictive pericarditis (primary distinguishing factor for restriction vs. constriction).

- Arrows point to dip and plateau (square root sign) seen in both restriction / constriction
  - Related to rapid equalization of atrial / ventricular pressures in early diastole
    - Majority of ventricular filling occurs in early diastole

CARDIAC TAMPONADE

- Hemodynamics
  - High pressure pericardial fluid compresses the heart and increases filling pressures throughout diastole → blunted y descent (in contrast to constriction / restriction)
  - Equalization of RV / LV end diastolic pressures and mean RA / LA pressures

- Pulsus paradoxus → > 10 mmHg fall in SBP during inspiration
  - Inspiration increases systemic venous return and right heart volumes
  - Under normal circumstances, RV free wall expands into the unoccupied pericardial space
  - In tamponade, the RV cannot expand into the pericardial space and the increased RV volume is accommodated by shifting the interventricular septum to the left → decreased LV diastolic volume and stroke volume
  - Also seen in constrictive pericarditis though the main mechanism is ↓ PV–LA driving pressure

- ○ Echocardiographic findings
  - ● RA diastolic collapse (seen during V systole)
  - ● RV diastolic collapse
  - ● Exaggerated MV / TV flow variation with respiration
    - > 25% inspiratory reduction in transmitral E velocity consistent with tamponade / constrictive pericarditis

RIGHT ATRIAL PRESSURE WAVEFORMS

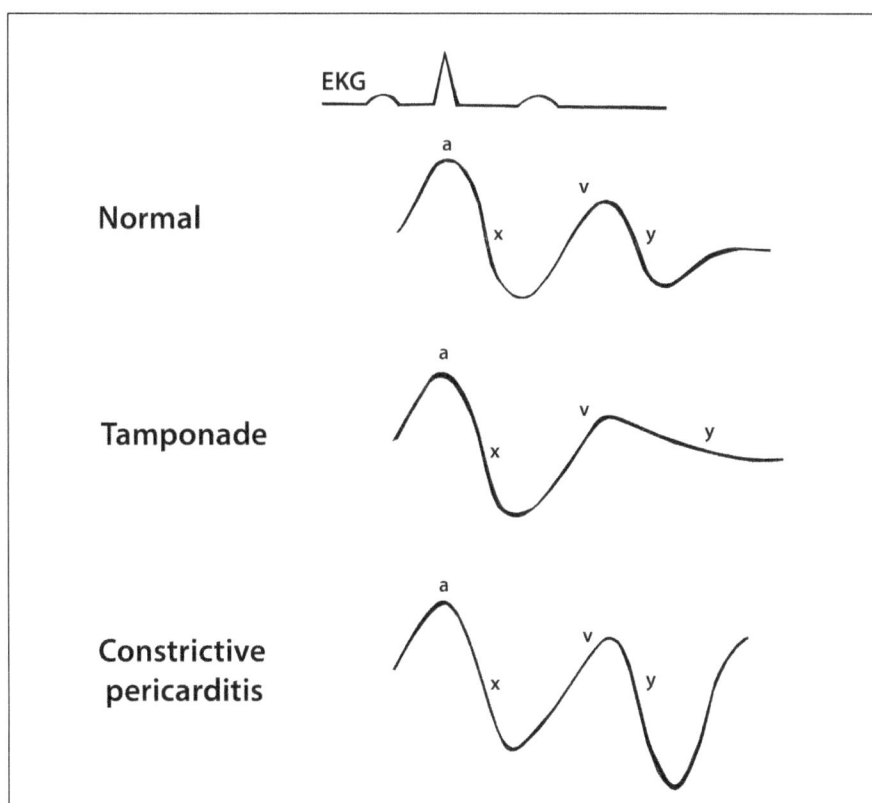

Figure 20.2 Right atrial pressure waveforms. *Note:* Blunted y descent seen in tamponade versus the steep y descent indicative of constrictive pericarditis / restrictive cardiomyopathy.

- Passive filling is minimal in tamponade due to equalization of diastolic pressures (blunted y descent)
- Most RV filling occurs via atrial systole with rapid equalization of pressures (steep × descent)

○ Abnormal compliance in constriction / restriction → rapid early diastolic filling with rapid equalization of atrial / ventricular pressures (steep y descent)

ACUTE PERICARDITIS

○ Treatment
- NSAIDs × 14 days
  - Ibuprofen 800 mg tid or indomethacin 80 tid or ASA 650 daily
  - Always use ASA post-MI due to increased risk of aneurysm formation with ibuprofen or indomethacin
- Colchicine 1–2 mg load / 0.5–1.0 mg daily × 3 months
- Steroids should be avoided in all but most refractory / recurrent cases as steroids increase risk for recurrent pericarditis and future constriction

REFERENCES

1. Seward JB, Casaclang-Verzosa G. Infiltrative cardiovascular diseases: Cardiomyopathies that look alike. *J Am Coll Cardiol.* 2010;55(17):1769–1779. (doi: 10.1016/j.jacc.2009.12.040)

2. Adler Y, Charron P, Imazio M, et al. 2015 ESC guidelines for the diagnosis and management of pericardial diseases. *Eur Heart J.* 2015;36(42):2921–2964. (doi: 10.1093/eurheartj/ehv318)

3. Geske JB, Anavekar NS, Nishimura RA, et al. Differentiation of constriction and restriction: Complex cardiovascular hemodynamics. *J Am Coll Cardiol.* 2016;68:2329–2347. (doi: 10.1016/j.jacc.2016.08.050)

4. Garcia MJ. Constrictive pericarditis versus restrictive cardiomyopathy? *J Am Coll Cardiol.* 2016;67:2061–2076. (doi: 10.1016/j.jacc.2016.01.076)

5. Talreja DR, Nishimura RA, Oh JK, Holmes DR. Constrictive pericarditis in the modern era: Novel criteria for diagnosis in the cardiac catheterization laboratory. *J Am Coll Cardiol.* 2008;51:315–319. (doi: 10.1016/j.jacc.2007.09.039)

6. Oh JK, Hatle LK, Seward JB, et al. Diagnostic role of Doppler echocardiography in constrictive pericarditis. *J Am Coll Cardiol.* 1994;23(1):154–162. (doi: 10.1016/0735-1097(94)90514-2)

7. Welch TD, Ling LH, Espinosa RE, et al. Echocardiographic diagnosis of constrictive pericarditis: Mayo clinic criteria. *Circ Cardiovasc Imaging.* 2014;7(3):526–534. (doi: 10.1161/CIRCIMAGING.113.001613)

8. Hatle LK, Appleton CP, Popp RL. Differentiation of constrictive pericarditis and restrictive cardiomyopathy by Doppler echocardiography. *Circulation.*1989;79(2):357–370. (doi: 10.1161/01.CIR.79.2.357)

9. Lange RA, Hillis LD. Clinical practice. Acute pericarditis. *N Engl J Med.* 2004;35(21):2195–2202. (doi: 10.1056/NEJMcp041997)

CHAPTER 21

PERIOPERATIVE CARDIOVASCULAR EVALUATION AND MANAGEMENT

SURGICAL RISK CATEGORIES

- Low risk (< 1% risk of MACE)
  - Endoscopy
  - Cataract
  - Breast biopsy

- Elevated risk (> 1% risk)
  - Aortic or other major vascular surgeries
  - Intraperitoneal / intrathoracic
  - Carotid endarterectomy / head and neck
  - Orthopedic
  - Prostate

- Current guidelines no longer make a distinction between intermediate- and high-risk procedures since both are treated similarly in terms of preoperative management

SURGICAL RISK FACTORS

- Major risk factors
  - Unstable angina
  - Decompensated heart failure
  - Myocardial infarction within the last 30 days
  - Significant arrhythmia
  - Significant valvular disease

- Intermediate risk factors
  - Stable angina
  - Prior MI > 30 days
  - Compensated CHF
  - Diabetes
  - Chronic renal insufficiency (CR > 2.0)

PREOPERATIVE WORKUP

- Emergency surgery → OR

- Active symptoms / conditions, nonemergent surgery → treat the active issues and reconsider surgery when stable

- Low-risk surgery / asymptomatic → OR (**regardless of risk factors)**
  - Preoperative ECG carries a **Class III** indication for asymptomatic patients undergoing low-risk surgery

- Functional capacity ≥ 4 METs / asymptomatic → OR **regardless of risk factors**

- No risk factors → OR **regardless** of functional capacity or surgical risk category

- 1+ risk factor / elevated risk surgery
  - **Consider** noninvasive testing only if it will alter management

KEY POINTS

○ Low-risk surgery → OR

○ No risk factors → OR

○ Functional capacity ≥ 4 METs → OR

○ Only strict indication to **consider** noninvasive testing preoperatively = 1+ risk factor **and** elevated risk surgery

○ Indications for revascularization are identical to patients not anticipating surgery
  ● Left main > 50%
  ● 3 vessel disease
  ● 2 vessel disease (including proximal LAD) and EF < 50% or ischemia on imaging
  ● Unstable angina / NSTEMI / STEMI
  ● High-risk findings on noninvasive imaging (see Chapter 2: Chronic CAD)

PERIOPERATIVE MANAGEMENT OF ANTIPLATELET AGENTS POST-PCI

○ Aspirin should **not** be stopped for any elective surgery

○ Nonurgent surgery should be delayed 4–6 weeks after balloon angioplasty or bare metal stent placement

○ P2Y12 inhibitor may be discontinued 6 months after DES for nonurgent surgery (Class I)
  ● May consider discontinuation of P2Y12 after 3 months when the risk of delaying surgery outweighs the risk of stent thrombosis

REFERENCES

1. Fleisher LA, Fleischmann KE, Auerbach AD, et al. 2014 ACC/AHA guideline on perioperative cardiovascular evaluation and management of patients undergoing noncardiac surgery: A report of the American College of Cardiology/American Heart Association Task Force on Practice Guidelines. *J Am Coll Cardiol.* 2014;64:e77–137. (doi: 10.1016/j.jacc.2014.07.944)

2. Boersma E, Kertai MD, Schouten O, et al. Perioperative cardiovascular mortality in noncardiac surgery: Validation of the Lee cardiac risk index. *Am J Med.* 2005;118:1134–1141. (doi: 10.1016/j.amjmed.2005.01.064)

3. Patel AY, Eagle KA, Vaishnava P. Cardiac risk of noncardiac surgery. *J Am Coll Cardiol.* 2015;66(19):2140–148. (doi: 10.1016/j.jacc.2015.09.026)

4. Patel MR, Dehmer GJ, Hirshfeld JW, Smith PK, Spertus JA. ACCF/SCAI/STS/AATS/AHA/ASNC 2009 appropriateness criteria for coronary revascularization: A report of the American College of Cardiology Foundation Appropriateness Criteria Task Force, Society for Cardiovascular Angiography and Interventions, Society of Thoracic Surgeons, American Association for Thoracic Surgery, American Heart Association, and the American Society of Nuclear Cardiology. *Circulation.* 2009;119:1330–1352. (doi: 10.1161/CIRCULATIONAHA.108.191768)

5. Banerjee S, Angiolillo DJ, Boden WE, et al. Use of antiplatelet therapy/DAPT for post-PCI patients undergoing noncardiac surgery. *J Am Coll Cardiol. 2017*;69(14):1861–870. (doi: 10.1016/j.jacc.2017.02.012)

6. Levine GN, Bates ER, Bittl JA, et al. 2016 ACC/AHA guideline focused update on duration of dual antiplatelet therapy in patients with coronary artery disease: A report of the American College of Cardiology/American Heart Association Task Force on Clinical Practice Guidelines. *J Am Coll Cardiol.* 2016;68:1082–1115. (doi: 10.1016/j.jacc.2016.03.513)

CHAPTER 22

ESSENTIAL CARDIOVASCULAR MANIFESTATIONS AND CARE OF RHEUMATOLOGIC DISEASES

Cardiac manifestations of rheumatologic diseases are vast, but will make up a small proportion of the ABIM exam. The table in this chapter highlights the key elements necessary for diagnosis and treatment of each disease process.

Table 22.1 Key Elements for Diagnosis and Treatment of Diseases

Disease	Clinical Findings	Diagnosis	Cardiac Manifestations	Treatment
Lyme Disease	Circular rash with central clearing (erythema migrans) / arthralgias	Lyme antibody by Western blot	Various degrees of AV block	Doxycycline or ceftriaxone
Rheumatoid Arthritis	• Autoimmune arthritis • Joint destruction	Rheumatoid factor	• Pericarditis • Myocarditis • Increased incidence of CAD / MI	Steroids +/– immunomodulators
Systemic Lupus Erythematosus	• Multiple organ systems affected • Arthritis and skin manifestations most common	• Antinuclear antibody (ANA) • Anti-Smith • Anti-DS-DNA • Anticardiolipin antibody • Lupus anticoagulant	• Pericarditis • Valvulitis / Libman-Sacks endocarditis → sterile vegetation • Myocarditis	• Pericarditis → NSAIDs / steroids for refractory symptoms • Valvulitis → anticoagulation if thrombotic events occur • Myocarditis → steroids

Giant Cell Arteritis	• Fever • Headache • Visual changes • Jaw claudication	Temporal artery biopsy	• Aortitis • Vasculitis • Vascular stenoses (including coronaries)	Steroids
Ankylosing Spondylitis	Chronic pain and stiffness in the low back and buttocks	HLA-B27	Aortic insufficiency	Symptomatic treatment
Systemic Sclerosis (Scleroderma)	Thickening of skin, especially of face, hands, and feet	Clinical diagnosis	• Pulmonary hypertension • Pericardial disease • (Effusions / pericarditis / constriction)	Symptomatic treatment

Disease	Clinical Findings	Diagnosis	Cardiac Manifestations	Treatment
Sarcoidosis	Restrictive pulmonary physiology → shortness of breath	• FDG PET • Biopsy → noncaseating granulomas	• Conduction disease • Ventricular arrhythmias • Sudden death	• Steroids • PPM / ICD may be necessary for advanced conduction system disease or ventricular arrhythmias
Kawasaki Disease	• Initial viral type illness • Rash on hands and feet • Mucosal involvement	Clinical diagnosis	Coronary artery aneurysms → increased thrombosis risk later in life	IVIG

Takayasu's Arteritis	• Females • Asian ancestry • < 40 years old • Acute illness followed by vasculitis	Clinical diagnosis	• Large vessel vasculitis → Stenosis or aneurysm • **Classic lesion is long, smooth, subclavian stenosis**	Steroids
Still's Disease	• Cyclic fever • Rash • Arthritis • Hepatitis	Clinical diagnosis	Pericarditis	Steroids
Churg-Strauss Syndrome (eosinophilic granulomatosis with polyangiitis)	• Asthma • Eosinophilia	• ANCA + • Skin biopsy → leukocytoclastic vasculitis with eosinophilic infiltration	• Heart failure → Eosinophilic myocarditis • Valvular disease	Steroids + cyclophosphamide or rituximab

REFERENCES

1. Wormser GP, Dattwyler RJ, Shapiro ED, et al. The clinical assessment, treatment, and prevention of Lyme Disease, Human Granulocytic Anaplasmosis, and Babesiosis: Clinical practice guidelines by the Infectious Diseases Society of America. *Clin Infect Dis*; 2006 43(9):1089–1134. (doi: 10.1086/508667)

2. Miloslavsky EM, Stone JH. Chapter 31: Cardiac manifestations of rheumatologic diseases. In: Gaggin HK, Januzzi, JL. *MGH cardiology board review*. London: Springer London; 2013:515–523. (doi: 10.1007/978-1-4471-4483-0)

3. McEvoy M, Murphy JG. Chapter 83: Systemic disease and the heart. In: Murphy JG, Lloyd MA. *Mayo clinic cardiology concise textbook*. 3rd ed. Rochester: Mayo Scientific Press; 2007:1017–1026.

4. Rogers BA, Rimmerman C. Chapter 54: Effects of systemic diseases on the heart and cardiovascular system. In: Griffin BP, Rimmerman CM, Topol EJ. *The Cleveland clinic cardiology board review*. Philadelphia: Lippincott Williams & Wilkins; 2007:713–721.

CARDIAC MANIFESTATIONS OF ENDOCRINE DISEASE

HYPERTHYROIDISM / THYROTOXICOSIS

- ↓ TSH / ↑ T3/T4
- Tachycardia / increased sympathetic tone
- Afib is common
  - No indication to cardiovert when thyrotoxicosis is present
- Treatment
  - Beta-blockers
  - Methimazole
  - PTU for thyroid storm

HYPOTHYROIDISM

- ↑ TSH / ↓ T3/T4
- Dry skin / periorbital puffiness / delayed deep tendon reflexes / fatigue

- ↓ cardiac output / ↑ systemic vascular resistance / pericardial effusion
- Myxedema coma
  - Altered mental status (often comatose) / hypothermia / bradycardia / hypotension
  - Treatment
    - IV levothyroxine / hydrocortisone 100 mg IV q8h

ADRENAL INSUFFICIENCY

- Primary cardiac manifestations: cardiomyopathy, CHF, hypotension
- Primary adrenal insufficiency (Addison's disease) → glucocorticoid and mineralocorticoid deficiency
  - ↓ cortisol / ↑ ACTH
    - Confirm with ACTH stimulation
      - Give 250 mcg ACTH → cortisol less than 18 mcg/dL = Addison's disease
  - Treatment
    - Glucocorticoids (hydrocortisone or prednisone) and mineralocorticoids (fludrocortisone)
- Secondary → ACTH deficiency
  - ↓ cortisol / ↓ ACTH

CUSHING SYNDROME

- Excess cortisol secretion due to adrenal adenomas or ACTH-producing pituitary adenomas
- Easy bruisability / proximal muscle weakness / hirsutism
- Hyperkalemia / systemic hypertension / LVH
- Typically treated with surgical resection of adenoma

PHEOCHROMOCYTOMA

- Catecholamine-secreting tumor
- Episodic severe systemic hypertension / palpitations / cardiomyopathy
- Diagnosis
  - Initial screen with plasma metanephrines
  - Confirm with 24-hour urinary catecholamines and metanephrines
    - If positive, image to localize location of the tumor
- Treatment
  - Surgical resection
    - Alpha (phenoxybenzamine) / beta-blocker prior to surgery

PRIMARY ALDOSTERONISM

- Systemic hypertension / hypokalemia
- Diagnosis
  - Aldosterone-to-renin ratio (ARR)
    - ARR ≥ 20 **and** plasma aldosterone concentration ≥ 15 ng/dL
      - Plasma renin activity usually < 1.0 ng/dL
  - Confirm with sodium or fludrocortisone suppression test
    - Positive → perform adrenal CT
      - Unilateral disease → perform adrenal vein sampling to prove functioning adenoma (incidentalomas are common)
- Treatment
  - Unilateral disease → surgical resection
  - Bilateral disease → medical management
    - Aldactone / low-sodium diet

ACROMEGALY

- Pituitary tumor → growth hormone excess
- Systemic HTN / CHF
- HTN treated with diuretics and sodium restriction / conventional therapies for CHF

PRIMARY HYPERPARATHYROIDISM

- Excess parathyroid hormone → hypercalcemia
- Systemic HTN / short QT

REFERENCES

1. McEvoy M, Murphy JG. Chapter 83: Systemic disease and the heart. In: Murphy JG, Lloyd MA. *Mayo clinic cardiology concise textbook.* 3rd ed. Rochester: Mayo Scientific Press; 2007:1017–1026.

2. Rogers BA, Rimmerman C. Chapter 54: Effects of systemic diseases on the heart and cardiovascular system. In: Griffin BP, Rimmerman CM, Topol EJ. *The Cleveland clinic cardiology board review.* Philadelphia: Lippincott Williams & Wilkins; 2007:713–721.

3. Wei NJ, Pallais JC. Chapter 32: Cardiovascular disease in endocrine disorders. In: Gaggin HK, Januzzi JL. *MGH cardiology board review.* London: Springer London; 2013:524–532. (doi: 10.1007/978-1-4471-4483-0)

4. Chrousos GP. Hyperaldosteronism workup. Retrieved April 20, 2017 from http://emedicine.medscape.com/article/920713-workup#c8

CHAPTER 24

HYPERLIPIDEMIA

○ Cholesterol is essential component of cell membranes / steroid hormones / bile acids

○ Lipids packaged / transported in lipoproteins made up of:

  ● Triglyceride core / phospholipid shell / free cholesterol

  ● Specialized apolipoproteins provide structural support / receptor recognition

   • Lp(a) confers increased CHD risk independent of LDL

   • Apo(a) may interfere with plasminogen → prothrombotic

  ● Routine assessment of Lp(a) and / or Apo(a) is **not** recommended

LIPOPROTEIN TRANSPORT PATHWAYS

- ○ Intestinal pathway → transport dietary triglycerides (TG) to liver / peripheral tissue
  - ● Dietary TG packaged with APO B48 and cholesterol to form chylomicron
    - Lipoprotein lipase hydrolyzes chylomicron → releases FFA, used by skeletal muscles, other organs
    - Chylomicron remnant taken up, degraded by liver

- ○ Hepatic pathway → transports TG / cholesterol between liver / peripheral tissues
  - ● TG / cholesteryl esters packaged in liver with Apo B100 to form VLDL
  - ● Lipoprotein lipase hydrolyzes VLDL → releases FFA to peripheral tissues → produces LDL (predominantly cholesterol) → degraded in the liver via LDL receptor (recognizes Apo B100) or deposited in blood vessel walls to form foam cells

STATINS

- ○ HMG-CoA reductase inhibitors → blocks rate limiting step of sterol synthesis
  - ● → increased expression of hepatic LDL receptors
  - ● → enhanced plasma clearance of LDL
  - ● → decreased VLDL production
    - Risk of myositis increased with concomitant fibrate (esp. gemfibrozil) / niacin use
    - Lovastatin / simvastatin / atorvastatin metabolized via CYP3A4
      - ○ Caution with macrolides / antifungals / cyclosporine / verapamil / amlodipine / ranolazine / grapefruit juice
    - Statins contraindicated in pregnancy (Class X)

FIBRATES

○ Inhibit APO B and VLDL production

○ Drug of choice for hypertriglyceridemia

MAJOR NON-LDL RISK FACTORS

○ Smoking

○ HTN

○ Low HDL (< 40-year-old male / < 50-year-old female)

○ FH premature CAD (< 55-year-old male / < 65-year-old female)

○ Age (> 45-year-old male / > 55-year-old female)

TREATMENT RECOMMENDATIONS

○ Estimate 10-year ASCVD risk every 4–6 years

○ Treatment goal no longer to specific LDL value

○ Treatment goal based upon statin intensity
  - High-intensity statin → goal LDL reduction ~ 50%
    • Atorvastatin 40–80 mg
    • Rosuvastatin 20–40 mg
  - Moderate-intensity statin → goal LDL reduction ~ 30%–50%
    • Atorvastatin 10–20 mg
    • Rosuvastatin 5–10 mg
    • Simvastatin 20–40 mg
    • Fluvastatin 40 mg
    • Lovastatin 40 mg
    • Pravastatin 40–80 mg

○ Measure LFTs prior to initiating statin / no indication to routinely check CK

○ Recheck lipids 4–12 weeks after change / initiation of statin

○ Four groups with Class I indication for statin:
  1. Clinical disease
     ● CAD / PVD / stroke / TIA
       • Age ≤ 75 → high-intensity statin
       • Age > 75 → moderate-intensity statin
  2. LDL ≥ 190
     ● High-intensity statin
  3. DM / age 40–75 / LDL 70–189
     ● Moderate intensity statin
     ● 10-year ASCVD risk > 7.5% → consider high-intensity statin
  4. Age 40–75 / LDL 70–189 / 10-year risk ≥ 7.5%
     ● Moderate- or high-intensity statin

PCSK9 INHIBITORS

○ Upregulate cellular LDL receptors → decreased circulating LDL

○ Indications
  ● Adults with homozygous or heterozygous familial hypercholesterolemia who require additional LDL lowering despite maximal tolerated statin dose or statin intolerance
  ● Clinical atherosclerotic disease requiring additional LDL lowering (typically defined as LDL > 100) on maximum therapy or statin intolerance

○ No clear outcome data to date

GENETIC DYSLIPIDEMIAS

- ○ Familial hypercholesterolemia
  - ● Autosomal dominant
  - ● LDL receptor mutation → increased circulating LDL levels
    - • **Tendon xanthomas** (especially achilles)
  - ● Homozygotes with LDL 400–1000
    - • Treated with plasmapheresis
  - ● Heterozygotes with LDL 190–350
    - • Treated with combination therapy

- ○ Familial defective APO B
  - ● Autosomal dominant
  - ● Defective APO B100 → reduced affinity for LDL receptor
  - ● Clinically indistinguishable from familial hypercholesterolemia
    - • Tendon xanthomas
  - ● Treatment is similar to familial hypercholesterolemia

- ○ Polygenic hypercholesterolemia
  - ● Common (1:20)
  - ● Combination of multiple genetic / environmental factors
  - ● LDL > 190 / **NO** xanthomas
    - • Typically normal TG (vs. familial combined)
  - ● Treat with combination therapy

- ○ Familial combined hyperlipidemia
  - ● LDL > 190 / TG > 300
  - ● Few clinical signs
  - ● Treat with combination therapy

- ○ Familial hypertriglyceridemia
  - ● Triglycerides 200–500
  - ● May be > 1000 in the context of ETOH / birth control pills / DM / hypothyroid
  - ● Treat with fibrate, niacin

REFERENCES

1. Stone NJ, Robinson J, Lichtenstein AH, et al. 2013 ACC/AHA guideline on the treatment of blood cholesterol to reduce athero-sclerotic cardiovascular risk in adults: A report of the American College of Cardiology/American Heart Association Task Force on Practice Guidelines. *Circulation.* 2014;129(25 suppl 2):S1–S45. (doi: 10.1161/01.cir.0000437738.63853.7a)

2. Nallamshetty S, Plutzky J. Chapter 6: Lipoprotein disorders. In: Gaggin HK, Januzzi JL. *MGH cardiology board review.* London: Springer London; 2013:105–119. (doi: 10.1007/978-1-4471-4483-0)

3. FDA Briefing Document. Endocrinologic and Metabolic Drugs Advisory Committee (EMDAC). June 10, 2015. Accessed September 29, 2017.

4. Myerson M. PCSK9 Inhibitors: A brief primer. Retrieved March 28, 2016 from http://www.medscape.com/viewarticle/861024#vp_1

CHAPTER 25

CARDIAC TUMORS

METASTATIC TUMORS

○ Metastatic disease is much more common than primary cardiac tumors
- Melanoma → most common to metastasize to the heart
- Breast / lung / hematologic are also common

MALIGNANT PRIMARY TUMORS

(Account for 25% of primary tumors)

○ Angiosarcoma
- Seen most frequently in the right atrium
- More common in men

○ Rhabdomyosarcoma
- Arise in any cardiac chamber
- Typically involves the pericardium via direct extension from the myocardium

○ Cardiac lymphoma
- Very rare

○ Primary cardiac malignancies are typically very aggressive

○ Therapy is typically only palliative

BENIGN PRIMARY TUMORS

(Account for 75% of primary tumors)

- Myxomas are the most common
  - Most commonly occur in the left atrium attached to the interatrial septum
  - Treated with surgical resection

- Lipoma
  - Most common is lipomatous hypertrophy of the interatrial septum
  - Surgical resection only if symptomatic

- Papillary fibroelastoma
  - Typically associated with left-sided heart valves, especially the aortic valve
  - Risk of embolization → neurologic complications
  - Surgical resection typically indicated to prevent embolization risk

BENIGN EXTRACARDIAC TUMORS

- Thymomas
  - Can invade the pericardium → tamponade

REFERENCES

1. Tan TC, Hung JW. Chapter 19: Tumors of the heart. In: Gaggin HK, Januzzi JL. *MGH cardiology board review.* London: Springer London; 2013:329–337. (doi: 10.1007/978-1-4471-4483-0)

2. Samara M, Griffin BP. Chapter 59: Cardiac neoplasms. In: Griffin BP, Kapadia SR, Rimmerman CM. *The Cleveland clinic cardiology board review.* Philadelphia: Lippincott Williams & Wilkins; 2013:866–875.

3. Gaasch WH, Vander Salm TJ. Cardiac tumors. Retrieved August 9, 2017 from https://www.uptodate.com/contents /cardiac-tumors#references

THERAPEUTIC HYPOTHERMIA

CURRENT GUIDELINES

○ Indicated for unconscious patients suffering out-of-hospital cardiac arrest (in-hospital arrest carries IIb indication)
  - Only indicated for patients remaining comatose following return of spontaneous circulation
  - No proven benefit in the setting of isolated respiratory arrest

○ Cooling should be initiated within 6 hours of the return of spontaneous circulation
  - Goal temperature 32–36°C
  - Shivering produces heat → may need sedation / paralysis

○ Goal MAP during cooling period > 80 mmHg
  - Hypertension may be additive to the neuroprotection of cooling
  - Use norepinephrine, if necessary, to achieve MAP goal

○ Bradycardia is common during during cooling and no treatment is necessary in the absence of other complications or evidence of hemodynamic instability

○ Begin rewarming 24 hours after **initiation** of cooling
  ● Rewarm over 8–12 hours / 0.3–0.5˚C / hour

EXCLUSIONS

○ Head trauma

○ Surgery within 14 days

○ Active infection

○ Active bleeding
  ● Anticoagulation / lytics are **not** a contraindication

REFERENCES

1. Callaway CW, Donnino MW, Fink EL, et al. Part 8: Post-cardiac arrest care: 2015 American Heart Association guidelines update for cardiopulmonary resuscitation and emergency cardiovascular care. *Circulation.* 2015;132(18 suppl 2):S465–482. (doi: 10.1161/CIR.0000000000000262)

2. Scirica BM. Therapeutic hypothermia after cardiac arrest. *Circulation.* 2013;127:244–250. (doi: 10.1161/CIRCULATIONAHA.111.076851)

CHAPTER 27

BIOSTATISTICS AND ESSENTIAL CALCULATIONS / VALUES

ESSENTIAL STATISTICS

- ○ True Positive = TP
- ○ True Negative = TN
- ○ False Positive = FP
- ○ False Negative = FN
- ○ Sensitivity → proportion with disease who have a positive diagnostic test
  - TP/TP+FN
- ○ Specificity → proportion without disease with a negative diagnostic test
  - TN/TN+FP
- ○ Sensitivity / specificity inversely related

- Highly sensitive test is best for **screening**
  - FN needs to be as low as possible and FP are not a significant concern when screening
- Highly specific test is best for **confirmation**
  - Minimum number of false positives
- Positive predictive value (PPV) → proportion with positive test who actually have the disease in question
  - TP/TP+FP
- Negative predictive value (NPV) → proportion with negative test who do not have disease
  - TN/TN+FN
- Accuracy → ability of a test to correctly differentiate between those with and without disease amongst all patients tested
  - TP+TN/TP+FP+TN+FN
- Prevalence → proportion of population with a defined condition
- Incidence → number of new cases in a given time frame
- Sensitivity / specificity are **not** affected by prevalence
- PPV / NPV / accuracy are all affected by prevalence
- Likelihood ratios define the probability of a given test result occurring in patients with disease to the probability of the same result in patients without disease

○ Positive Likelihood Ratio (LR+) → probability a patient with disease has a positive test
  ◦ Sensitivity/1-Specificity
    • Higher the LR+, more likely a positive test is due to true disease

○ Negative Likelihood Ratio (LR–) → probability that a patient with disease has a negative test result
  ◦ 1-Sensitivity/Specificity
    • More negative the LR-, more likely a negative test is a true finding
  ◦ LR > 1 associated with disease / LR < 1 associated with absence of disease
  ◦ LR near 1 has little clinical utility because it does not appreciably change post-test probability of presence or absence of disease

HYPOTHESIS TESTING

○ Null hypothesis → any observed difference is due to chance and a true difference does not actually exist
  ◦ **Alpha** level → threshold value for a difference between groups to be considered statistically significant, i.e., probability that a difference between groups is actually due to chance (type I error)
    • **Alpha** level typically 0.05

○ P value → probability of obtaining the observed results
  ◦ If the P value is less than the predetermined **alpha** level, the difference between groups is considered statistically significant and the null hypothesis is rejected

- ○ Errors
  - Type I error → demonstrated difference between groups is actually due to chance as opposed to a true difference
    - Results in accepting the null hypothesis when it is actually true (false positive)
  - Type II error → no difference identified between groups when one actually exists
    - Results in accepting null hypothesis when it is actually false (false negative)

- ○ Confidence Intervals → range of values in which the true value is likely to reside
  - 95% CI indicates that the true value will be outside this range 5% of the time

BASIC CALCULATIONS / VALUES

- ○ Shunts
  - $Qp : Qs = SAO_2 - MVO_2 / PVO_2 - PAO_2$
  - $MVO_2 = 3(SVCO_2) + (IVCO_2) / 4$
  - SaO_2 difference > 7 mmHg between SVC or RA and PA should prompt full sat run to exclude L → R shunt
  - Systemic arterial saturation < 93% with no other identifiable cause should raise concern for R → L shunt

- ○ Qp/Qs < 1.5 = small L → R shunt

- ○ Qp/Qs 1.5 – 2.0 = intermediate size shunt

- ○ Qp/Qs > 2.0 = large L → R shunt

- ○ Qp/Qs < 1.0 = → L shunt

- Simplified Gorlin formula
  - AVA = CO (L/min) / sq root of mean gradient (mmHg)
- Cardiac output measurement
  - Thermodilution method → saline injected as a bolus through proximal port of PA catheter
  - Thermistor in the distal PA port measures the temperature of blood over a duration of time → temperature curve from which a computer derives the cardiac output
    - Significant TR → injectate traverse back and forth across the tricuspid valve producing a curve consistent with a low flow state → falsely low CO calculation
    - AI, MR will also underestimate CO
  - Fick method → uses arterial-venous oxygen difference to determine oxygen extraction by the body and thereby calculate cardiac output
  - Thermodilution method most accurate in the setting of high output states
  - Fick method most accurate in the setting of low output states and irregular rhythms
- Normal pressures / values
  - Measure all values at end expiration

Table 27.1 Normal Pressures / Values

Pressure Measurement Site or Metric	Normal Pressure or Value
Right atrium	10 mmHg
Right ventricle	15–25 / 1–8 mmHg
Pulmonary artery	15–25 / 4–12 mmHg
Pulmonary capillary wedge pressure	4–12 mmHg (LA = LVEDP in absence of MV disease)
Left atrium	2–12 mmHg
Left ventricle	90–140 / 5–12 mmHg
Cardiac output	4-6 L/min
Cardiac index	2.4–4.0 L/min/m2
Systemic vascular resistance	700–1600 dynes / 9-20 Wood units
Pulmonary vascular resistance	20–130 dynes / 0.25-1.6 Wood units

Measure all values at end expiration

REFERENCES

1. Lauer MS, Gorodeski EZ. Chapter 7: Clinical epidemiology and biostatistics. In: Griffin BP, Kapadia SR, Rimmerman CM. *The Cleveland clinic cardiology board review.* Philadelphia: Lippincott Williams & Wilkins; 2013:55–63.

2. Szymonifka J, Healy BC. Chapter 13: Basic statistics. In: Gaggin HK, Januzzi, JL. *MGH cardiology board review.* London: Springer London; 2013:224–237. (doi: 10.1007/978-1-4471-4483-0)

3. Gami AS, Rihal CS. Chapter 3: Evidence-based medicine and statistics in cardiology. In: Murphy JG, Lloyd MA. *Mayo clinic cardiology concise textbook.* 3rd ed. Rochester: Mayo Scientific Press; 2007:55–60.

4. Hayden S, Brown M. Likelihood ratio: A powerful tool for incorporating the results of a diagnostic test into clinical decision making. *Ann Emerg Med.* 1999;33:575–580. (doi: 10.1016/S0196-0644(99)70346-X)

5. Harvey JE, Heupler FA. Chapter 45: Hemodynamic measurements. In: Griffin BP, Kapadia SR, Rimmerman CM. *The Cleveland clinic cardiology board review.* Philadelphia: Lippincott Williams & Wilkins; 2013:654–670.

6. Abtahian F, Jang IK. Chapter 9: Cardiac catheterization, coronary arteriography, and intravascular diagnostics. In: Gaggin HK, Januzzi, JL. *MGH cardiology board review.* London: Springer London; 2013:153–173. (doi: 10.1007/978-1-4471-4483-0)

7. Nishimura RA. Chapter 118: Invasive hemodynamics. In: Murphy JG, Lloyd MA. *Mayo clinic cardiology concise textbook.* 3rd ed. Rochester: Mayo Scientific Press; 2007:1393–1406.

CHAPTER 28

PHYSICAL EXAM ESSENTIALS

A large proportion of board question stems contain extensive physical examination details. A thorough grasp of physical examination findings is essential.

BASIC PRINCIPLES

- ○ Right-sided murmurs increase in intensity with inspiration
  - Lone exception is ejection sound associated with pulmonic stenosis → decreases with inspiration

- ○ Apical impulse
  - Noted in the 4th/5th intercostal space / medial to mid-clavicular line
  - Sustained → LVH
  - Widened / laterally displaced → LV dilation
  - Diffuse heave in left parasternal region → RVH

- ○ S1
  - Split → Ebstein's anomaly
  - Variable → afib
    - With regular rhythm → AV dissociation / clue to VT when associated with wide complex rhythm
  - Soft → LV failure / early MV closure in acute AI

- ○ S2
  - Aortic valve typically closes just before pulmonic valve
  - Physiologic splitting
    - Inspiration → increased right sided blood flow
      - ○ Longer RV ejection period → A2–P2 widening
      - ○ Shorter RV ejection with expiration → A2–P2 narrow
  - Fixed splitting → wide A2–P2, unchanged by respiratory cycle
    - **ASD**
    - RV failure
    - VSD with left-to-right shunt (due to early aortic valve closure)
  - Persistent splitting → A2–P2 remains split during expiration and widens further with inspiration
    - RBBB / pulmonary HTN / pulmonic stenosis (Delayed P2)
    - Severe MR / VSD (early A2)
  - Paradoxical splitting → typically due to delayed A2
    - P2 occurs before A2 with expiration / single sound with inspiration
      - ○ LBBB
      - ○ RV pacing
      - ○ HOCM
      - ○ Ischemia

- S3
  - Usually disappears by age 40
    - Normal in pregnancy
- S4
  - Produced by atrial contraction into a stiff ventricle
  - Left-sided S4 → aortic stenosis / HOCM / acute ischemia
  - Right-sided S4 → pulmonic stenosis / pulmonary HTN
- Continuous murmurs
- To be considered continuous must start in systole and continue **through** S2
  - Coronary fistula / pulmonary AV fistula / coarctation of the aorta
    - All radiate to the back
  - PDA
    - Heard best LUSB radiating to the left clavicle
    - Diastolic portion becomes shorter as pulmonary HTN progresses
    - Differential cyanosis seen with Eisenmenger's physiology
      - Cyanotic lower extremities with normally oxygenated upper extremities
  - Mammary souffle
    - Benign
    - Heard in late pregnancy / lactation
- Innocent murmurs
  - Soft
  - **Never** pansystolic
  - No other abnormal clinical findings

VALVULAR LESIONS

○ Aortic stenosis
  - Heard best at RUSB with radiation to the carotids
    - Murmur intensity decreases moving further up the neck vs. carotid bruit that gets louder higher in the neck
  - Delayed carotid upstroke / lo-w amplitude (pulsus parvus and tardus)
  - Murmur peaks later with increasing severity
  - A2 reduced or inaudible with severe AS / S2 may be paradoxically split
  - Aortic ejection sound consistent with bicuspid aortic valve

○ Aortic sclerosis
  - Early peaking / normal S2 / normal carotid upstroke

○ Supravalvular aortic stenosis
  - Carotid pulse discrepancy (R > L)
  - Right arm SBP > 10 mmHg higher than left arm
  - Normal S2

○ Aortic insufficiency
  - Peripheral signs
    - Hyperdynamic carotid pulse
    - Double peaked pulse
    - Femoral systolic BP > 40 mmHg > brachial artery (Hill sign)
  - Chronic AI → holodiastolic murmur
  - Acute AI → early diastolic murmur only
    - Due to rapid equalization of aortic / LV pressures
  - Murmur radiating to left sternal border / apex → consider leaflet abnormality
  - Murmur radiating to right sternal border → consider aortic root disease / dissection

- Mitral stenosis
  - Low-pitched, diastolic rumble heard best at the apex
    - Often with associated diastolic "opening snap" (OS)
  - A2–OS interval indicates severity
    - Left atrial pressure increases with worsening mitral stenosis
  - OS occurs earlier in diastole as LA pressure rises
    - A2–OS interval ↓ with increasing MS severity
    - OS intensity ↓ with increasing MS severity

- Mitral regurgitation
  - Heard best at the apex with radiation to the left axilla
  - Laterally displaced PMI
  - Posterior mitral valve leaflet pathology → murmur radiates to the aortic area
    - Differentiate from aortic stenosis by examining the carotids
      - MR will not radiate to the neck
  - Acute, severe MR only heard in early systole due to rapid equalization of LV–LA pressures

- Mitral valve prolapse
  - Systolic click
  - Increased preload / afterload → improved leaflet coaptation → click moves away from S1, closer to S2
    - Quieter / shorter murmur
  - Decreased preload / afterload → poor leaflet coaptation → click closer to S1
    - Louder / longer murmur

- Pulmonic stenosis
  - Right upper sternal border / crescendo / decrescendo
  - Radiates to left shoulder / back
  - Increases with inspiration
  - Diminished P2
  - Persistently split S2 (due to prolonged pulmonic ejection time)
  - Early ejection click
    - **Decreases** with inspiration
    - Moves closer to S1 with increasing severity of stenosis
  - Delayed murmur peak / widening of A2–P2 split with increasing severity

- Pulmonic regurgitation
  - Right upper sternal border
  - Increases with inspiration
  - Loud P2
  - Persistently split S2

- Tricuspid stenosis
  - Left lower sternal border / xiphoid
  - Increases with inspiration
  - Large a waves / blunted y descent on JVP

- Tricuspid regurgitation
  - Left lower sternal border / radiates to the right
  - Left parasternal lift
  - Large V waves

HEMODYNAMIC MANEUVERS

○ Handgrip – Increases afterload

○ Squatting – Increases preload

○ Standing – Decreases preload

○ Valsalva – Decreases preload

○ Post-PVC – Increases contractility

○ Amyl nitrate – ↓ afterload acutely followed by ↑ venous return (↑ preload)

Table 28.1 Effects of Hemodynamic Maneuvers on Murmur Intensity

	AS	HCM	MVP	MR	Explanation
Handgrip	↓	↓	↔	↑	↑ afterload
Squatting	↑	↓	↓	↑	↑ preload
Standing	↓	↑	↑	↓	↓ preload
Valsalva	↓	↑	↑	↓	↓ preload
Post-PVC		↑↑			↑ contractility
Amyl nitrate	↑	↑	↔	↓	↓ afterload / ↑ venous return

SPECIFIC CONDITIONS

○ Hypertrophic obstructive cardiomyopathy
  ● Murmur heard mid to lower left sternal border / harsh
  ● Distinguished from AS by hemodynamic maneuvers
  ● Rapid carotid upstrokes / sometimes bifid (spike and dome) → due to mid systolic ventricular outflow obstruction
  ● Paradoxical splitting of S2

- Atrial septal defect
  - RV heave
  - Increased P2
  - Fixed split S2
  - ↑ JVP
  - Mid systolic ejection murmur / pulmonary ejection click
    - Related to ↑ pulmonary blood flow
    - Diastolic tricuspid flow murmur also heard if large L → R shunt

- Ventricular septal defect
  - Holosystolic / will shorten with pulmonary HTN
  - Persistently split S2
  - Thrill at left sternal border

- Coarctation of the aorta
  - Radial – femoral pulse delay
  - Frequently occurs in association with bicuspid aortic valve

PREGNANCY

- Tachycardia

- Laterally displaced PMI

- Persistent split S2

- S3

- Systolic flow murmur

- Mammary souffle

- Peripheral edema

RA / JUGULAR VENOUS WAVEFORM

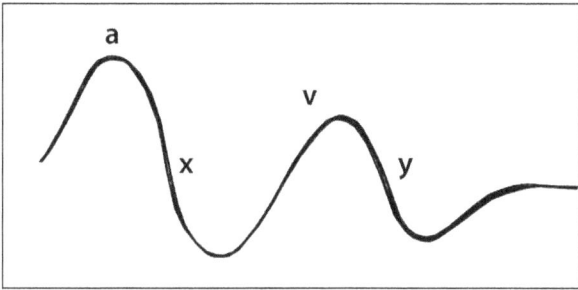

Figure 28.1   Normal RA / jugular venous waveform.

○ a – RA systole

○ x – RA relaxation / RV filling

○ c – RV contraction / protrusion of closed TV into RA

○ v – RV systole / RA filling with closed TV

○ y – RV diastolic filling

REFERENCES

1. Shub C. Chapter 1: Cardiovascular examination. In: Murphy JG, Lloyd MA. *Mayo clinic cardiology concise textbook.* 3rd ed. Rochester: Mayo Clinic Scientific Press; 2007:3–26.

2. Gaggin HK, Drachman DE. Chapter 1: History and physical examination. In: Gaggin HK, Januzzi JL. *MGH cardiology board review.* London: Springer London; 2013:1–22. (doi: 10.1007/978-1-4471-4483-0_1)

3. Asher CR, Bonilla Isaza CA. Chapter 2: Cardiac physical examination. In: Griffin BP, Kapadia SR, Rimmerman CM. *The Cleveland clinic cardiology board review.* 2nd ed. Philadelphia: Lippincott Williams & Wilkins; 2013:4–23.

4. Fang JC, O'Gara PT. Chapter 12: The history and physical examination: An evidence-based approach. In: Bonow RO, Mann DL, Zipes DL, Libby P, Braunwald E. *Braunwald's heart disease. A textbook of cardiovascular medicine.* 9th ed. Philadelphia: Elsevier Saunders; 2012:107–125.

PHARMACOLOGY ESSENTIALS

VAUGHAN WILLIAMS CLASSIFICATION

○ IA – Sodium-channel blockers / Lengthen action potential duration
  - Quinidine / procainamide / disopyramide

○ IB – Sodium-channel blockers / Shorten action potential duration
  - Lidocaine / mexiletine

○ IC – Sodium-channel blockers / Don't affect action potential duration
  - Flecainide / propafenone
    - **Always** coadminister with AV nodal blocking agent to reduce risk of 1:1 flutter

○ II – Beta-blockers

○ III – Potassium-channel blockers / prolong repolarization / lengthen QT
  - Amiodarone / sotalol / dofetilide / dronedarone

○ IV – Calcium-channel blockers

- ○ Use-dependant drugs have increased effects at higher heart rates
  - ● Seen especially with Class IC agents
  - ● Much more effective at converting atrial fibrillation / flutter to NSR
    - • Basis for "pill in the pocket" approach
- ○ Reverse-use dependence
  - ● Increased drug effects at slower heart rates
    - • Class III agents
  - ● More effective at maintaining NSR than converting
  - ● Increased risk of torsades de pointes at slower heart rates

ANTIARRHYTHMIC OPTIONS IN ATRIAL FIBRILLATION

- ○ Structurally normal heart → propafenone / flecainide / sotalol
  - ● Amiodarone as second-line agent due to toxic side effect potential
  - ● Dofetilide as second line agent due to higher proarrhythmic risk, complexity of initiation
- ○ LVH > 1.3 cm → amiodarone
- ○ CAD / normal LVEF → sotalol / dofetilide
  - ● Amiodarone second line
- ○ CHF (systolic or diastolic) → amiodarone / dofetilide

IMPORTANT DRUG EFFECTS / INTERACTIONS

○ Amiodarone
  ● Requires close monitoring for multiple potential toxic side effects
    • Baseline ECG, thyroid function tests (TFTs), liver function tests (LFTs), pulmonary function tests (PFTs), CXR
  ● Repeat TFTs, LFTs, every 6 months
  ● Repeat ECG, CXR yearly
  ● Repeat PFTs as needed based upon symptoms

○ Statins
  ● Inhibit HMG-CoA reductase → rate limiting step of cholesterol biosynthesis
    • Leads to increased hepatic LDL clearance / decreased hepatic VLDL production
  ● Reduce (10 mg) or avoid simvastatin with any of the following:
    • Antifungals
    • Erythromycin
    • Clarithromycin
    • HIV drugs
      ○ Low dose atorvastatin, pitavastatin, rosuvastatin are all appropriate options
    • Calcium-channel blockers
    • Amiodarone
    • Cyclosporine

○ ACE / ARB
  ● Renal failure, hyperkalemia

- Calcium-channel blockers
  - Dihydropyridine → nifedipine, amlodipine, felodipine
    - Lower extremity edema
  - Non-dihydropyridine
    - Diltiazem / verapamil
      - Negative inotropes / negative chronotropes
- Digoxin
  - Nausea, vomiting, diarrhea
  - Drowsiness, confusion, visual disturbance
- Thiazide diuretics
  - Gout / hypokalemia
- Hydralazine
  - Lupus-like syndrome
- Avoid nadolol / atenolol in renal failure
- Avoid metoprolol in hepatic failure
- Heparin
  - Heparin-induced thrombocytopenia
    - Fall in platelet count > 50% coinciding with heparin administration
    - **Do not** transfuse platelets
    - No warfarin until platelets return to normal
    - Increased risk for arterial thrombosis

COMMON VASOACTIVE DRUGS

Table 29.1 Common Vasoactive Drugs

Drug	Receptor	Effect
Phenylephrine	α	↑ afterload
Isoproterenol	β1 / β2	↑ HR / ↑ contractility / ↓ afterload
Norepinephrine	α > β1	↑ afterload / ↑ contractility
Epinephrine	β1 / β2 / α	↑ contractility / ↑ afterload
Dobutamine	β1 > β2	↑ contractility / ↓ afterload
Dopamine	4–10 mcg/kg/min → β1 > 10 mcg/kg/min → α	↑ contractility ↑ afterload
Nitroprusside	Arterial > venous dilator	↓ preload / ↓ afterload
Nitroglycerin	Venous > arterial dilator	↓ preload / ↓ afterload
Hydralazine	Arterial dilator	↓ afterload
Phentolamine	α antagonist	↓ afterload / ↑ contractility / ↑ HR
Furosemide	Diuretic	↓ preload
Milrinone	Phosphodiesterase inhibitor	↑ contractility / ↓ afterload / ↓ pulmonary vascular resistance

REFERENCES

1. Karwacki Sheff EJ, Januzzi JL. Chapter 33: Pharmacology. In: Gaggin HK, Januzzi JL. *MGH cardiology board review.* London: Springer London; 2013:533–534. (doi: 10.1007/978-1-4471-4483-0_1)

2. Fuster V, Ryde'n LE, Cannom DS, et al. 2011 ACCF/AHA/HRS focused updates incorporated into the ACC/AHA/ESC 2006 guidelines for the management of patients with atrial fibrillation: A report of the American College of Cardiology Foundation/ American Heart Association Task Force on Practice Guidelines. *Circulation.* 2011;123:e269–e367. (doi: 10.1161/CIR.0b013e318214876d)

3. Salter BS, Weiner MM, Muoi A. Trinh MA, et al. Heparin-induced thrombocytopenia: A comprehensive clinical review. *J Am Coll Cardiol.* 2016;67:2519–2532. (doi: 10.1016/j.jacc.2016.02.073)

4. Ou NN, Oyen LJ, Jahangir A. Chapter 111: Cardiac drug adverse effects and interactions. In: Murphy JG, Lloyd MA. *Mayo clinic cardiology concise textbook.* 3rd ed. Rochester: Mayo Clinic Scientific Press; 2007:1291–1308.

5. Vassallo P, Trohman RG. Prescribing amiodarone: An evidence-based review of clinical indications. *JAMA.* 2007;298(11):1312–1322. (doi: 10.1001/jama.298.11.1312)

www.ingramcontent.com/pod-product-compliance
Lightning Source LLC
Chambersburg PA
CBHW070720220326
41598CB00024BA/3242